The Dysl Handbook 2001

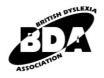

Published by

The British Dyslexia Association

98 London Road

Reading

RG1 5AU

Helpline: 0118 966 8271

Administration: 0118 966 2677

Web Site - http://www.bda-dyslexia.org.uk/

ISBN 1-872653-31-6

9 781872 653310

The British Dyslexia Association

The British Dyslexia Association aims to ensure that there is a way forward for every dyslexic person, so that he or she receives proper teaching, help and support, and is given an equal opportunity to achieve his or her potential in order to lead a fulfilled and happy life.

The Dyslexia Handbook 2001

A compendium of articles, checklists, resources and contacts for

dyslexic people, their families and teachers. The Dyslexia Handbook

is substantially updated and revised each year.

Edited by

Ian Smythe

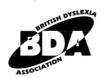

Published by

The British Dyslexia Association

Editorial note

The views expressed in this book are those of the individual contributors, and do not necessarily represent the policy of the British Dyslexia Association.

The BDA does not endorse the advertisements included in this publication.

Whilst every effort has been made to ensure the accuracy of information given in this handbook, the BDA cannot accept responsibility for the consequences of any errors or omissions in that information.

In certain articles the masculine pronoun is used purely for the sake of convenience.

British Dyslexia Association
    The Dyslexia Handbook 2001
    1. Great Britain. Education
    I. Title II. Ian Smythe
ISBN 1 872653 31 6

Published in Great Britain 2001
Copyright © The British Dyslexia Association 2001

Designed and typeset by Ibis Creative Consultants Ltd, 34 Collingwood Road, Sutton, Surrey SM1 2RZ
Tel: 0208 770 0888
Fax: 0208 770 0936
Cover photographs by Ian Smythe, Ibis Creative Consultants Ltd

The British Dyslexia Association
98 London Road, Reading RG1 5AU

Telephone: 0118 966 2677
Helpline: 0118 966 8271
Fax: 0118 935 1927
E-mail: Helpline: info@dyslexiahelp-bda.demon.co.uk
           Administration: admin@bda-dyslexia.demon.co.uk

Website: http://www.bda-dyslexia.org.uk/

Registered Charity Number: 289243
Registered in England no. 1830587

Contents

Part 1 - The British Dyslexia Association and other organisations helping dyslexic people

This section deals with organisations in the UK and around the world which work towards a better future for all dyslexic people.

Part 2 - About dyslexia

This section tells you about dyslexia, its causes and how to recognise it. It also explains about some of the related specific learning difficulties a dyslexic person may experience.

Directory (blue pages)

This section contains details of local dyslexia associations and other organisations from whom you can get help and support. Also listed are details of independent schools with special provision for dyslexic pupils, teacher training centres, dyslexia-related Internet sites and other useful contacts.

Part 3 - Managing dyslexia

This section contains chapters on ways to cope with dyslexia, whether you are a parent, a teacher or a dyslexic person in the adult world; on obtaining special provision for dyslexic children; and suggestions for further reading.

Part 4 - Around dyslexia

This section contains chapters on other conditions which in some cases are found to occur together with dyslexia.

Chair's Address

It is an honour and a challenge for me to take over as Chair of
the BDA as it enters the new Millennium. I salute its past
achievements, made possible by cooperative action of
associations, staff, corporate members, teachers, volunteers,
parents, trustees and my predecessor, Nick Monck.

The BDA enters the new Millennium with great clarity of
purpose and a determination to succeed. Its objectives span
the full dyslexia age range. We want increasingly to Catch Em
Young, before lack of confidence begins to bite; we want every
school to become dyslexia friendly; and every LEA, FE college
and university to recognise the need for appropriate support
and to provide it. Already many have made changes in policy
and educational practice; and we especially welcome them as
supporting corporate members.

We are also calling for a better deal for dyslexic adults. This
year sees the launch of a concerted campaign for greater
awareness and understanding of the many adults whose
dyslexia is only discovered later in life and of those who simply
do not realise that they are dyslexic. The BDA believes that
knowing is important. It is only when you understand your
dyslexia that you can find the right way forward for you,
whatever your age.

The BDA's programme of action includes easily accessible
assessment of adult dyslexia; adult learning programmes based
on a full understanding of dyslexia; basic skills tutors with the
specialist qualifications necessary to teach dyslexic adults;
advice centres which provide information in a dyslexia friendly
format and – last but not least – encouraging employers to
develop and implement dyslexia friendly policies.

We have already shown that dyslexia friendly schools would be better for every pupil. The challenge now is to win the argument in the wider world. Not only gaining greater support for dyslexic people, but also highlighting the different ways of looking at problems that they bring to the worlds of work and education. We need to harness the creativity and instinct for innovation and problem solving of people with dyslexia in the interests of a rapidly changing ideas-based economy, as well as in their own. People with dyslexia need understanding to overcome their difficulties, but equally society and the economy need their potential.

I hope that this handbook will contribute to building the awareness and understanding necessary to help unlock the full potential of every dyslexic child, young person and adult. Last year's version certainly helped me learn rapidly about dyslexia, the issues and the providers.

Please stay in touch with the BDA. We produce a range of useful publications. For a small amount of money, you can help our work to make a real difference for dyslexic people. Not just this year, but as we go forward into the century. Will you join us (see page 22 for details) or send a donation today?

Kirsteen Tait

Chair, British Dyslexia Association

Editor's introduction

In this edition 2001, I would like to think that once again we have an exciting list of contributions, with something for everybody. Of particular interest is the Special Section on whole school approach by Neil MacKay, and I am delighted that he will be taking on the role of editor next year. But first I will explain that this is my third and last edition as editor, as I believe that it is important for the growth of the Handbook that new editorial views are brought in.

So as I step back, I would like to reflect a little on what has happened over recent years, and more importantly, where I believe we still have to go, in both the short and long term.

As a relative newcomer to the scene (only 15 years) I do not have the experience of others, but having had mentors like the late Marion Welchman, as well as the like of Steve Chinn and Tim Miles, I have found myself increasingly concerned about the gap between what is supposed to be in place and what is actually there.

The 1989 UN Rights of the Child says that all children have the right to education. I believe that should be changed. It should say the every child has the right to **appropriate** education. That, in effect, is what the Code of Practice sets out to achieve. So where, in my opinion, does it go wrong?

There are many areas one could highlight, but my main concern is assessment.

Repeatedly the Code of Practice suggests that assessment should be carried out by appropriate, normed, tests. But where are those tests?

If we agree that in order to successfully remediate the dyslexic individual we have to have an effective measurement of their cognitive profile, then my question is where is that tool? Yes, there are a number of commercially available tests, but who will recommend them, and will they lead to effective remediation, or just another label? Will they cover all aspects, or are they the result of narrow research? And who pays?

But beyond that there is the question of who will do that assessment? Why do I repeatedly encounter frustrated teachers who are not sure of what test to use, how to administer it and interpret and use the information? Why does it often take 18 months before an Educational Psychologist (EP) can be called in? And even then the EP may be frustrated by a lack of direction on what instruments to use.

So what is the way forward?

The answer is simple, the implementation is more difficult! Let us start by developing an assessment procedure that can be used by teachers so that they can at least have an indication of where the problems lie, and implement immediately an appropriately structured IEP. Let us have it peer group reviewed (researchers, educational psychologists and teachers!) and easy to use. And let's have it distributed FREE to ALL schools. But let's also have TRAINING in how to use such a test.

To do this we do not have to re-invent the wheel, but simply recognise what needs to be done, and find the will to fund it. Only then, I believe, will the Code of Practice have any real meaning.

Ian Smythe

Part 1 - The British Dyslexia Association and other organisations helping dyslexic people

Part 1 - The BDA and other organisations

A summary of BDA activities

On behalf of its members the mission of the BDA is:

• to present its policies to government, politicians and national policy making agencies in the fields of education, employment and access to employment and the providers of goods and services to secure improvement for people with dyslexia

• to provide support to local associations, supporting members and individual members through the provision of effective services - such as helplines, befriending, computer advice and information and development

• to provide training for befrienders and other volunteers

• to produce publications for professionals and for general awareness

• to support member organisations directly through attendance at their events, through joint events and projects, and through continuing dialogue about their needs

• to encourage, monitor and disseminate research.

The British Dyslexia Association - Who we are and what we do

Joanne Rule, in her role as Chief Executive of the BDA, gives a brief tour of the BDA, its activities and its members.

The BDA is the voice of dyslexic people. The charity offers advice, information and help to dyslexic people, their families and the professionals who support them. Alongside this practical help, we are working to raise awareness and understanding of dyslexia and to effect change. The BDA is made up of 97 local dyslexia associations, together with 116 supporting corporate members. Together we form one of the world's leading dyslexia organisations and a channel for all the latest thinking and research on the subject. The charity believes that dyslexia must be seen as a combination of both abilities and difficulties. These difficulties can be significantly reduced by early intervention and appropriate support.

National Helpline

The BDA's National Helpline (0118 966 8271) is our main link to the community. Last year the charity received more than 126,000 web site, telephone, email and written enquiries.

Our affiliated local associations also operate helplines giving detailed information about what is available in their area, in terms of services both to dyslexic people and to anyone with an interest in dyslexia. See the Directory (blue pages) for local helpline numbers. Many associations provide a wide range of support and training services as well as opportunities to network with others similarly involved with dyslexia.

Befrienders

The BDA supports a national network of highly motivated and trained volunteers known as befrienders, whose aim is to enable parents to get the right help for their child. Call your local dyslexia association to make contact with a befriender who can help you.

Early identification

Working closely with health care professionals and parents, the BDA promotes the early identification of dyslexia in pre-school children. In partnership with AFASIC, the speech impairment charity, the BDA has produced a multidisciplinary training package for health professionals, nursery workers and all those working in the early years. This work was funded by Glaxo Wellcome and undertaken by the Department of Human Communication Science, University College London.

Education

Our aim is to ensure that teachers are able to recognise dyslexia and to take suitable action. We work very closely with schools, local authorities and other relevant bodies at nursery, primary, secondary, further and higher education levels. We also provide support to teachers, governors and special needs coordinators through a wide range of publications and conferences. The BDA Accreditation Board sets the criteria for, and supports, specialist teacher training programmes at universities and other teacher training establishments, leading to the award of Associate Membership of the BDA (AMBDA) and Approved Teacher Status (ATS) for school teachers. There are equivalent awards for support tutors working in further and higher education institutions. There is also an award (ALSA) for Learning Support Assistants. We strongly endorse the need for in service training in special needs for mainstream teachers and, although we are primarily concerned with children in state education we also work closely with the independent sector. The BDA is campaigning for the spread of "dyslexia friendly schools".

Adults

Recent years have seen a growth in support groups for dyslexic adults, although much remains to be done. To encourage this development, the BDA has produced guidelines on setting up support groups for dyslexic adults.

The BDA offers information to students in further and higher education and to all dyslexic adults about employment issues and continuing education. We highlight both the needs and the talents of dyslexic people in the workplace, urging employers to create pathways to literacy and to develop an understanding of the contribution made by dyslexic adults.

Influencing public policy and provision

As well as supporting dyslexic individuals - and their families - the BDA works with Government and national agencies to put in place the policies that will help the professionals to deliver lasting improvements for dyslexic people.

Membership of the BDA

There are two main classes of membership of the BDA: affiliated local dyslexia associations and supporting members, known as corporate members.

Affiliated local associations

Local dyslexia associations support families on the ground. Joining your local dyslexia association will be a real help to you and to others.

Local dyslexia associations are usually registered charities in their own right, with their own constitutions, membership and managing committees.

Most charge an annual membership subscription which varies from one association to another. When a local association affiliates to the BDA, part of that subscription is paid to the BDA. Three times a year every local member receives the magazine Dyslexia Contact. Local associations also receive regular bulletins from the BDA about current issues, may send representatives to the Council of the BDA, and are represented on its Local Associations Board.

Supporting Corporate membership

Supporting Corporate members provide educational or specialist dyslexia services or undertake research into dyslexia. They join the BDA because they support its aim to make government departments, local education authorities, corporations and the public at large aware of the difficulties and strengths of dyslexic people and to spread information and understanding.

They support advances in the education of dyslexic people and the dissemination of the results of research into dyslexia.

Communicating across the network

Computer advice service

Through a national network of coordinators, supported by an expert volunteer computer committee, we help parents and dyslexic adults to draw the maximum benefits that computers and educational software can offer. We also publish a range of helpful booklets and fact sheets.

Publications

In addition to this handbook, the BDA produces many other publications including three issues a year of the magazine, Dyslexia Contact which is available on subscription and sent to all members of affiliated local associations, and a comprehensive range of booklets and leaflets. See the list on page 294 for further details.

Conferences and exhibitions

The BDA organises conferences for families, school governors and professionals at both local and national levels as well as a prestigious international conference every three years, the next being scheduled for April 2001. The BDA is represented at many of the major education exhibitions and often leads seminars.

Internet website

The BDA operates a web site on the Internet which provides information about events, useful resources and has links to other international sites.

Visit us at: http://www.bda-dyslexia.org.uk/

E-mail: Helpline: info@dyslexiahelp-bda.demon.co.uk

Admin: admin@bda-dyslexia.demon.co.uk

Mailing subscription

The BDA mailing list is designed to keep you up to date with the latest news and developments in the world of dyslexia at a level that suits your needs.

Parent/Carer   £30 per year (£25 if paid by direct debit)
Subscribers to the Parent/Carer mailing list will receive:
3 mailings per year
Inclusions:
Handbook (1 per year - in the January mailing)
BDA Contact Magazine (3 issues per year)
BDA Publications and Resources lists
Events lists

Dyslexic Adult   £30 per year (£25 if paid by direct debit)
3 mailings per year
Inclusions:
Adult Introduction Pack
Handbook or any other BDA publication (1 per year – included in the January mailing)
BDA Contact Magazine (3 issues per year)
BDA Publications and Resources lists
Events lists

Educator/ Professional   £70 per year (£60 if paid by direct debit)
6 mailings per year
Inclusions:
All those for Parent/Carer, plus:
ICT update (3 mailings per year)
Concessionary rates at selected conferences
Key publication – The BDA has a publication to cover dyslexia at every age. When BDA selects a key title it will be sent to you free of charge.

Institution/ Commercial	£130 per year 10 mailings per year As for Parent/Carer and Educator/ Professional plus: Dyslexia Journal. International research and practice (4 issues per year)
Dyslexia Journal	£35 per year. International research and practice (4 issues per year)
Overseas	Subscription outside the UK carry an extra annual charge to cover the increased costs of despatch.
Corporate Membership	If you would like to receive an application form for corporate membership please write to the BDA address below.

Rates valid until 31 December 2001.

Your support is vital to effect change for dyslexic children, young people and adults.

A donation to the BDA will make a real difference. If you are a UK tax payer why not make your donation worth substantially more by signing the Gift Aid declaration on page 23 (below the Direct Debit Form).

Address your application form or Direct Debit mandate, or donation, or request more information to:

BDA, 98 London Road, Reading RG1 5AU.

Photocopy as required

BDA Membership form

Please complete this form and the direct debit instruction overleaf if applicable and post to: BDA, 98 London Road, Reading RG1 5AU.

Name ....

Address..

....

Postcode ....Tel: .... Fax: ....

SUBSCRIPTIONS

Parent/Carer	Annual subscription	£30	❏
	Direct Debit subscription	£25	❏
Dyslexic adult	Annual subscription	£30	❏
	Direct Debit subscription	£25	❏
Educational/ Professional	Annual subscription	£70	❏
	Direct Debit subscription	£60	❏
Institution/ Commercial	Annual subscription	£130	❏
Dyslexia Journal		£35	❏
Overseas	subscriptions carry an additional annual charge to cover postage	£10	❏
Donation	Here is my gift of If you are a UK taxpayer please also complete the Gift Aid declaration opposite	£............	
Total	Please enter the total amount	£	

Method of payment: cheque ❏   Direct Debit (see opposite) ❏

Card Number _ _ _ _   _ _ _ _   _ _ _ _   _ _ _ _   Expiry date _ _   _ _

Issue No/Valid From: _____

Signature: _____ Today's date: _____

To make an instant donation please call 0118 966 2677 and quote your credit/debit card details.

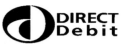

Instruction to your Bank or Building Society to pay by Direct Debit

Please fill in the whole form using a ballpoint pen and send it to:

BRITISH DYSLEXIA ASSOCIATION
98 London Road
Reading
RG1 5AU

Originators Identification Number

4	0	2	5	1	5

Name(s) of Account Holder(s)

Reference Number

Instruction to your Bank or Building Society
Please pay the BRITISH DYSLEXIA ASSOCIATION Direct Debits from the account detailed in this instruction subject to the safeguards assured by the Direct Debit Guarantee.
I understand that this instruction may remain with the BRITISH DYSLEXIA ASSOCIATION and, is so, details will be passed electronically to my Bank/Building Society.

Bank/Building Society account number

Bank Sort Code

To the manager	Bank/Building Society
Address	
	Postcode

Signature
Date

Bank and Building Societies may not accept Direct Debit Instructions for some types of accounts

✂ ---

Gift Aid

I would like the British Dyslexia Association to reclaim tax on any donation or membership subscriptions that I make. I have paid an amount of UK income tax or capital gains tax equal to any tax deducted.

Full Name _____ Date _____

Signature _____

Supporting Corporate Members of the BDA

The Supporting Corporate Members of the BDA continue to offer a variety of products and services to the membership in addition to their role in organising collaborative ventures. Here Paul Stanley, Chairman of the Supporting Corporate Members committee, looks at recent activities.

Activities of the Corporate Members Committee

The Government through the DfEE continues to make a steady stream of new initiatives and to publish a range of discussion documents. As a result, there continues to be a lot of activity in the special needs world and a continuing need for the BDA to represent the needs of the dyslexic individual. Supporting Corporate Members make a valuable contribution towards such representations and work closely with the BDA to ensure that the rights of the dyslexic individual are protected. Some of the key issues in which they have been involved recently include:

- The BDA/DI review

- The proposed new Code of Practice

- The placement of children with Statements of Special Educational Needs in independent schools

- Changes to 'A' Level entry gate issues

- The formation of a BDA professional committee

- Providing conferences for educational professionals, parents and the public at large

- Providing support and In-Service training for teachers of dyslexic pupils

- Promoting research and identifying appropriate assessment systems

About Supporting Corporate Membership

Since the initiatives taken to widen Supporting Corporate Membership, I am delighted to announce that applications have continued to come from a variety of sources and that membership almost totals 120. Membership falls into the following categories:

• Independent schools

• Mainstream schools or units

• Further and Higher Education

• Health

• Research institutions

• Commercial organisations

Supporting Corporate Members are entitled to:

• Copies of bulletins (the BDA Newsletter) and the magazine Dyslexia Contact

• Complementary annual Dyslexia Handbook and discount on subsequent copies

• The information and computer technology mailing

• Option to subscribe to the professional Dyslexia Journal at a discounted rate

• A free copy of key BDA produced publications

• Entry in annual Dyslexia Handbook, BDA web and other relevant BDA publications

• Discounts on selected BDA conferences, attendance and/or exhibition space

• E-mail circulation of BDA information and the option to join BDAFORUM

Supporting Corporate Members of the BDA support advances in the education of dyslexic pupils and the dissemination of the results for research into dyslexia. They support the BDA's aim to make Government Departments, Local Education Authorities, employers and the public at large aware of the difficulties and strengths of dyslexic people and to spread information and understanding.

As the initiatives to widen Supporting Corporate Membership have taken effect, the Supporting Corporate Members committee have discussed in detail the rotation of committee members in order to reflect the changing membership. The aim is that membership should be proportional according to the different membership criteria. Membership of the committee will be constantly evaluated and reviewed in order to reflect the constituent membership.

Supporting Corporate Members Open Day

Continuing the theme of representing greater width of membership, the Supporting Corporate Members Open Day for the year 2000 is planned (at the time of writing) to take place at the St George Sixth Form Centre site, City College, Birmingham. The agreed provisional programme includes the transition to Further Education, careers support and appropriate ICT resources. The opportunity to examine issues to do with Further Education and the needs of dyslexic students in terms of careers support and ICT resources has been welcomed by all Supporting Corporate Members.

The role of Chairman

As the current Chairman, I continue to work closely with the Supporting Corporate Members committee, Joanne Rule (Chief Executive, BDA) and the BDA staff to further advance the cause of the dyslexic individual in today's society. I am currently co-opted onto the management board of the BDA. With so many new proposals and the publication of many discussion documents, these are exciting times. If you are interested in joining us, get in touch with the BDA and add your voice to the cause.

Paul Stanley is Chairman of the BDA Supporting Corporate Members Committee and Headmaster of Appleford School.

For further details about the activities and membership of the Supporting Corporate Members, please contact the BDA, 98 London Road, Reading, RG1 5AU.

Some key dates in 2001

Just a few of the BDA's planned events are outlined below. For further details contact the BDA head office on 0118 966 2677. Local dyslexia associations and independent dyslexia centres also hold events all year round. Check the directory pages for contact numbers to find out what's on in your area or check our website

http://www.bda-dyslexia.org.uk/

Jan 10-13   BDA stand and seminars at BETT 2001 Grand Hall, Olympia, London

Mar 22-24   BDA stand and seminars at the Education Show, NEC, Birmingham

April 18-21   BDA International Conference, York

May 22-23   BDA stand at Special Needs North

May 24-25   Welsh Education Show, Cardiff

June   BDA Spellbound Ball, London

Oct/Nov   Dyslexia Awareness Week

Nov 1-3   BDA stand at Special Needs Exhibition, London

Nov 17   Annual General Meeting

BDA WEBSITE
www.bda-dyslexia.org.uk/

The Dyslexia Institute
Shirley Cramer, Executive Director

The Dyslexia Institute is the largest provider of teaching and assessment services for individuals with dyslexia in the UK. From small beginnings in 1972 the Institute now has a nationwide network of 24 Centres and 132 teaching outposts. In addition the Institute runs accredited training courses, develops educational materials and has undertaken a multi-year research project to provide a scientific evaluation of multi-sensory teaching.

Assessment and Specialist Teaching

Under the supervision of our Department of Psychology the DI assesses approximately 7000 children and adults annually. Some 75 educational psychologists work for the DI on a consultancy basis and receive regular training on the latest assessment tools and techniques to ensure a standard national service for individuals and families.

All the Centres offer individual and small group teaching and full assessments, but many of the Centres also now work closely with their local education authorities and other government agencies to train teachers and improve understanding about the needs of people with dyslexia.

The DI, whose head office is in Staines, currently employs 230 specialist teachers who teach over 3000 students a year ranging in age from 5 to 69. The majority of our students are school-aged children who are struggling in school and need the specialised help of the Institute.

All students work on an individual programme, catering to their particular needs. Some may be taught in a "duo" with one other pupil or with two others in a "trio". Our aim is to create independent learners who are able to cope effectively in school or work.

The Dyslexia Institute Literacy Programme and Units of Sound Multimedia tool are the two core programmes used by our teachers. Our recently published Dyslexia Institute Maths Programme is popular with the teachers as is the Study Skills Programme.

Teacher Training

The Training Service of the Institute has been developing new courses in response to the need to train more specialist teachers. This year the DI is running a two year Post Graduate Diploma and a one-year PG certificate which may be studied live or by distance learning. York University validates these courses. Our new courses are part funded by the Teacher Training Agency and we had an excellent report as a result of the DI's first OFSTED inspection. An application for BDA accrediation for the new courses has been made.

The DI runs a programme of INSET courses in schools for specialist and mainstream teachers and parents. These courses have been helpful to teachers involved in implementing the National Literacy and Numeracy Strategies. Many of our short courses are sponsored by companies and trusts and done in partnership with local education authorities.

Educational Development

The DI has made evaluation of its work a high priority and is constantly looking at ways to improve and streamline its services and its educational tools. The latest Units of Sound CD rom is now available and is appropriate for Key Stage 3 through to adult. This is an easy to use multimedia learning

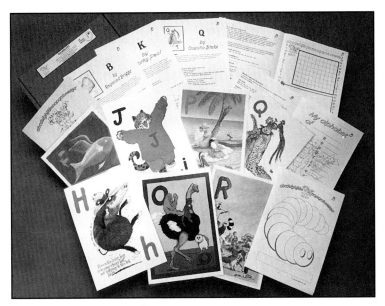

Abracadabra A.B.C.

Resource Pack for teachers

26 wonderful, stimulating Alphabet pictures by well known children's book illustrators. For each letter Abracadabra provides a 'talk-about' section, worksheets and creative ideas for using the pictures with students with a range of abilities. The pack was developed by and is sold by the Dyslexia Institute.

resource. Last year's Active Literacy Kit, designed to provide the essential foundations for literacy for children who have not yet begun to read, has been widely welcomed. The DI Trading Company will distribute our educational materials.

Staff at the DI are provided with regular in-service training to ensure quality and up to date services throughout the organisation. The progress of our students is monitored closely.

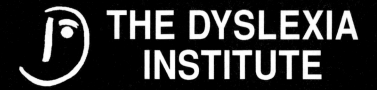

Research: the Spell-it Project

The Spell-it project (Study Programme to Evaluate Literacy Learning through Individualised Tuition) is the Institute's most ambitious research project to date, designed to evaluate the effects of structured programmes of intervention for 7 year old pupils who are experiencing specific difficulties in learning to read, write and spell. This multi-year Intervention is being conducted in partnership with the Centre for Reading and language Studies at the University of York and involves working closely with local education authorities around the country. The project is being funded by the National Lotteries Charities Board, The Department for Education and Employment, WH Smith and the Institute's Bursary Fund.

The study investigates the differences between dyslexic students who have received structured intervention and those who have not. The project links together recent scientific progress with the experience of working with children with dyslexia. The ultimate objective of the research is to develop cost-effective programmes of support that can be tailored to the type and severity of literacy difficulty. A key aspect of the project is the development of materials and a programme of support that parents can use with their children at home. This Home Support Programme will also be evaluated. The results of this long-term research will help us and others in the field to provide better help for dyslexic individuals in the future.

Helping Students with Few Resources

The Institute raises funds to support students and their families who cannot afford the fees for tuition. The Dyslexia Institute Bursary Fund (DIBF) now provides funding for 10% of our students and the demand for this help is increasing each year.

"As I See It" Competition

The DI and the BDA work alongside each other in complementary ways to help individuals with dyslexia. The collaboration exists at a national and a local level. For the second year the BDA has joined forces with the DI in the promotion of the As I See It competition, which has been running for 16 years. The competition enables the dyslexic individual of all ages to showcase their artistic or writing talents. The results show the innate strengths of the dyslexic individual.

For details of all our centres and services contact our head office at:

The Dyslexia Institute

133 Gresham Road

Staines

Middlesex TW18 2AJ

Phone: 01784 463851 or visit our Website at:

WWW.dyslexia-inst.org.uk

5th BDA International Conference

DYSLEXIA:
At the Dawn of the New Century

University of York
18–21 April 2001
Chair: Professor Rod Nicolson

Cutting edge research will be at the heart of this dynamic and exciting conference, which will celebrate the successes of past decades whilst also looking to the future.

Dyslexia now has official government recognition. Children can be screened for the condition in their earliest years. Adult needs are beginning to be recognised and addressed. Advances have been made in terms of scientific discovery; technology has really taken off. Yet there is still much work to be done.

This conference will present the very latest research, whilst looking at best practice for teachers, psychologists, learning support assistants, policy makers and relevant others.

Further details and updates will be found at the conference main website at:
www.bdainternationalconference.org

The Hornsby International Dyslexia Centre

The Hornsby International Dyslexia Centre continues to improve its services, as well as extend its international appeal. Here, Jonathan Dixon, Chief Executive, looks at an exciting development in this past year as well as what they now offer.

The Hornsby Centre has always been involved in the international forum. Last year we sent a team to South Africa and Zimbabwe. This year (2000) saw the first of the The Hornsby International Workshops which sought to take the Hornsby experience to another context. The workshop, carried out on behalf of the Hong Kong Education Department in Hong Kong, took the form of a two week course, designed not only to get across the information, but also to work with the local professionals to improve the awareness, recognition and remediation of dyslexia. The five members of the Hornsby team delivered a course based around a series of workshops to 30 key personnel who would also teach others the technique learnt during the course. Each of the workshops took an aspect of dyslexia and discussed and modified it to the local context. These workshops varied from creating the Chinese vocabulary for dyslexia (e.g. finding the right word for phonological discrimination) to discussing the phonics method of learning English (in Hong Kong children start learning English at age 5, using a rote method similar to the way of learning Chinese characters). Shorter courses were also held in both Brazil and Bulgaria, both aimed at raising the awareness and understanding of dyslexia.

For many years the Hornsby Centre was based at Glenshee Lodge, the home of its founder Bevé Hornsby, and in very recent times ran its attendance courses in offices in Balham.

We have been very fortunate to have acquired from Wandsworth Council a building near to Clapham Junction station where all our activities can be housed in a single location. We moved in early in September and despite a few teething problems we have settled into our new home very well. We would welcome visitors to view our facilities.

The Hornsby Centre itself was set up in 1984 by Bevé Hornsby to continue the teacher training course that she set up with Frula Shear in 1973 when Bevé was the Head of the Speech Therapy Clinic at Bart's Hospital. It was Bevé and Frula who wrote Alpha to Omega now in its 5th edition.

Today the Hornsby Centre is a registered charity whose aims are :

- to advance education by training teachers and students to teach dyslexics

- to advance the education of persons suffering from dyslexia and to alleviate the difficulty

- to advance the education of the public about the incidence, effect and remediation of dyslexia

- to initiate or co-operate in research into such incidence, effects or treatment and publish the results thereof.

In the achievement of these aims the Hornsby Centre offers the following facilities:-

- Attendance courses: OCR Diploma and Certificate, Hornsby Diploma and Hornsby Foundation Course.

- Distance Learning Course: Hornsby Diploma or Hornsby Diploma at Post Graduate level.

- Bookshop stocked with a wide range of text books, workbooks and equipment concerning specific learning difficulties and teaching the dyslexic individual.

- A regularly published Newsletter distributed to Friends of the Centre

- Update Conferences covering topical issues

- Assessments

- Maintains a list of Tutors who are able to offer one to one tuition

- Provides bespoke courses both within the UK and overseas

- Some funding of research associated with special educational needs and specifically dyslexia

The Hornsby International Dyslexia Centre welcomes approaches from other organisations and is willing to co-operate with them in all areas.

For details of new developments and courses run by the Hornsby International Dyslexia Centre contact us at :

The Hornsby International Dyslexia Centre
Wye Street
London SW11 2HB

Tel: 020 7223 1144

Fax: 020 7924 1112 or

E-mail: dyslexia@hornsby.co.uk

Website: www.hornsby.co.uk

The Helen Arkell Dyslexia Centre

As the Centre celebrates its 30th anniversary as the country's oldest dyslexia organisation and charity in 2001 and welcomes its new Executive Director, Rosie Wood, following the retirement of Gail Goedkoop in August 2000. Peter Smith looks back at events of the past 30 years and forward to the future.

On April 26th 1971, 30 years ago, Helen Arkell opened the doors for the first day of The Helen Arkell Dyslexia Centre, helped by Joy Pollock and Elizabeth Waller. This was the culmination of Helen Arkell's pioneering work for the dyslexia movement which she embarked on during the 1950's and 60's and for which she was awarded the MBE, and which helped pave the way for the other national dyslexia organisations which soon followed.

The Centre was initially based in Fulham Road, London. Within a few months Helen had also opened the Centre at Frensham in what had been the old stable block of her grandparents' home. With more space and car parking available at Frensham, this was developed as the headquarters and the London centre was eventually closed.

Helen remained as Head of Centre until 1979 when Joy Pollock, who had been deputy head from the beginning, took over the reins. Joy retired when the London centre closed in 1987 and Gail Goedkoop was appointed Director.

During her 13 years as Director, Gail, who had previously been the Courses Director, guided the Centre through a long period of sustained growth and development that continues today. Her particular interest has always been in professional training for teachers and she introduced a wide range of new courses and qualifications and enabled thousands of teachers and classroom assistants to gain expertise in teaching children and adults with specific learning difficulties. She was also very involved in the development and accreditation of awards offered by the British Dyslexia Association and the Royal Society of Arts, now the OCR, a very important role for the Centre that has been taken over by Bernadette McLean, the Academic Director.

Continuing the tradition of appointing from within, Rosie Wood took over as Executive Director on Gail's retirement in August 2000. Rosie had been an Assistant Director and Head of Speech and Language.

The original plan in 1971 was that the Centre should be a specialist teaching establishment – which it still is. However there was so great a demand from other teachers to learn the specialist skills that within months Helen had started the first ever professional training course. These also quickly spread to Frensham where they were first held in the village hall. Also, 30 years ago there were no formal assessment procedures and of course many psychologists and educators strongly resisted the existence of dyslexia. Helen and her helpers found themselves having to devise their own assessment methods. Thus the three key activities of assessment, tuition and professional training came together in a very short time and remain the core services some 30 years later.

Today the Centre provides probably the widest range of services of any organisation of its type and is highly regarded for its professional expertise and the quality of its care and support for individuals. The latter has always been the single most important aspect of its strategy and philosophy; the need to maintain it is the main reason why the Centre has always decided against opening in other parts of the country.

Services are available for both the individual with dyslexia and related specific learning difficulties and for the educational community, in line with the Centre's mission of maximising educational opportunity for people of all ages and making available the most effective methods of recognition and treatment of these difficulties throughout the community. Staff work to build partnerships at all levels – individual, school, Local Authority.

Services for individuals include consultations, assessment, tuition, speech and language therapy, study skills, social skills and counselling. All initial consultations are free and are aimed at enabling people to decide the course of action most appropriate for their child or themselves. The Centre provides some 500 free consultations each year and is unique in providing this service. In most cases a consultation is followed by an assessment. Assessments are carried out by educational psychologists, specialist teachers and speech and language therapists. They cover literacy, numeracy and speech and language. Well over 1,000 full assessments, examination certificates and needs assessments for the Disabled Students Allowance are carried out each year.

Specialist tuition is carried out by over 100 specialist teachers on a one-to-one basis for over 500 pupils of all ages at any one time. The Centre firmly believes that this is the only effective way of helping people with such diverse learning difficulties. Tuition is backed up by speech and language therapy and study skills where needed. Help with motivation and self-esteem is provided through counselling and social skills courses.

Recent new activities include summer schools which concentrate on study skills and social interaction, and a very busy mail order book and resources sales enterprise.

Key to much of the Centre's work is the Bursary Fund which is available for people who cannot afford the fees. Bursaries are available for all services. The Fund depends entirely on fundraising.

Right from the start in 1971, Helen Arkell recognised the importance of training teachers and helping schools – which she calls the `ripple effect'. This extends from individual teachers to whole schools to entire Local Authorities. Last year over 200 classroom assistants and teachers, at primary, secondary and FE/HE levels, trained on the Centre's Foundation (CLANSA), Certificate and Diploma courses in specific learning difficulties. One day courses in specialist topics such as NLP, thinking skills and assessment are also available to teachers. Bursaries are available to classroom assistants and teachers from state schools to help with training fees.

Services for schools and colleges start with Inservice training and awareness days – last year staff provided Inservice to over 50 schools across the country, from Teeside to Taunton. The next stage is the School Partnership Scheme, a 2 year programme aimed at transferring the Centre's skills to an entire school, and finally partnerships with Local Education Authorities. The Centre is currently working with Sutton Education Authority on a 3 year programme with all the schools in the Authority. School and LEA Partnerships are jointly funded by the Centre from grants from trusts, and by the school or LEA.

The Centre's annual national conference for teachers is a well established tradition, attracting delegates from all over the UK and overseas. The first was held in Oxford 25 years ago, and they now alternate between Cambridge and the Frensham area. Well known keynote speakers, often from the USA, cover topical themes in a practical, hands-on way.

Thanks to the work of people like Helen, the Centre and many others, people with dyslexia now enjoy an equality of opportunity that would have seemed incredible in 1971. All schools have SENCo's, there are special needs policies and codes of practice, appeal procedures, extra time for examinations, grants for IT equipment for HE students, PCs and laptops, a mass of special needs software, high general awareness and acceptance of dyslexia as a disability, strong media support and protection under the Employment Discrimination Act.

Despite these great advances, the need for organisations like The Helen Arkell Dyslexia Centre remains as strong as ever, as resources for dyslexia are still inadequate to meet demand. The pioneering phase has gone and the emphasis for the future will be on the delivery of services that everybody can access. The Centre remains firmly committed to the principles that Helen Arkell established 30 years ago. They are to provide high quality services tailored to meet the total needs of each individual, to train as many teaching professionals as possible and to work in partnership with schools and Local Authorities in order to make the skills and resources needed to help people with specific learning difficulties widely available throughout the community.

The 2001 conferences are on Monday 19th February and Saturday 3rd March 2001 and will be held at Alton College. Themes will be Study and Thinking Skills, and Social Interaction.

For further information about The Helen Arkell Dyslexia Centre and its services:

Tel: 01252 792400 or

Fax: 01252 795669.

www.arkellcentre.org.uk

Email general_enquiries@arkellcentre.org.uk

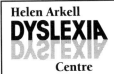

Scottish Dyslexia Association

The Scottish Dyslexia Association (SDA) is the leading dyslexia organisation in Scotland. Amongst the many other services provided, the SDA and its and its network of affiliated local branches aim to raise awareness of the nature of dyslexia and how it can affect children, young persons, and adults in all aspects of their daily life.

The SDA provides a service which is unique in Scotland giving advice, information and support to dyslexic people, their families, teachers, employers and to other professionals who have an interest in dyslexia.

A confidential telephone helpline service is in operation, manned by experienced knowledgeable staff. The helpline is open Monday to Friday from 9.00 a.m. until 5.00 p.m. Outside these times there is a telephone messaging service.

On behalf of dyslexic people in Scotland the SDA responds to consultation documents issued by the Scottish Executive and aims to influence the educational policy of both central and local government. SDA representatives attend meetings of all manner of formal and informal bodies to ensure that the voice of dyslexics in Scotland is heard by those who should hear it.

For further details and help contact
    Scottish Dyslexia Association
    Stirling Business Centre,
    Wellgreen, Stirling, FK8 2DZ

Dyslexia Helpline (Scotland): 01786 446650
Fax: 01786 471235
E-mail: dyslexia.scotland@dial.pipex.com
Website: www.dyslexia.scotland.dial.pipex.com

International Dyslexia Association

The International Dyslexia Association (IDA - formerly The Orton Dyslexia Society) is a worldwide, non-profit scientific and educational organization dedicated to the study and treatment of the learning disability, dyslexia. Executive Director, J. Thomas Viall, provides this brief overview of activities. If you have any questions or wish to receive more information about IDA, you may e-mail the Executive Director at: jtviall@interdys.org.

Brief History

IDA was founded in 1949 and has been serving individuals with dyslexia, their families and professionals in the field for more than 50 years. It was established to continue the pioneering work of Dr Samuel Torrey Orton, a neurologist who was one of the first to postulate the neurobiological basis of dyslexia. Along with Anna Gillingham and Bessie Stillman, he also worked to develop effective teaching approaches for individuals with dyslexia. Since the founding of our organization, many multisensory, structured, sequential, systematic methods of language instruction have been developed based on Dr. Orton's work. We proudly continue his philosophy that children with dyslexia can and should learn how to read. IDA receives no government support. We are funded through private donations, membership dues, foundation grants, sale of publications, conferences and other development efforts. IDA has just begun a "capital campaign" to purchase its own headquarters building which will serve as a true "international center" for research, collaboration and distance learning. As of this writing, more than US$1,500,000 have been donated to the project.

The Membership

To fulfill our important mission, IDA has more than 13,000 active members in approximately 60 countries. IDA has 43 branches within North America and two National Affiliates in Israel and The Philippines. Since our name change to The International Dyslexia Association in 1997, we are prudently expanding our international structure and outreach. We are currently in discussions with several other dyslexia associations around the world to expand the National Affiliate program. Our branches hold at least four public events (conferences, seminars, training sessions, parent and adult support groups, etc.) per year. Branches also provide local information and referral services through networks with private and public schools, diagnosticians, tutors, physicians, researchers, parents and individuals with dyslexia. Our membership consists of people with dyslexia, their families, professionals in the field of dyslexia and volunteers who work together for the benefit of individuals with dyslexia. Members receive discounts on publications, conferences and workshops, as well as a subscription to our peer-reviewed journal, "Annals of Dyslexia," a quarterly magazine, "Perspectives" and a member newsletter.

The Services

In addition to membership and branch services, we offer information and referral services to the public. The headquarters of IDA is a clearinghouse of valuable information, responding to an average of 1500 - 2000 contacts each month. Our services include:

1) free information and referrals

2) a Web Site containing free information on dyslexia, bulletin boards, a "Kids Only" section and will soon be used for distance learning activities

3) many publications on dyslexia

4) an annual international conference that brings together experts in the field and individuals with dyslexia

5) funding for educational and medical research

6) participation in public awareness and public education initiatives

7) monitoring of and lobbying for federal legislation of interest to people with dyslexia

8) teacher training seminars and parent and adult support groups.

9) Legal advocacy to defend the rights of people with dyslexia and other learning disabilities

10) IDA has also adopted a 5 year plan to develop a national (USA) system to accredit specialized (LD) teacher training programs and schools for students with learning disabilities.

The Conference

Our Annual International Conference is attended by professionals and parents from around the world. Our conferences attract more than 3,000 attendees from various disciplines. We also offer conference scholarships to teachers to expand the scope and impact of our conference. Our 50th Anniversary Conference was held in the United States in Chicago, Illinois on November 3-6, 1999. Featured speakers were Dr. Reid Lyon of the National Institutes of Health, Dr. Howard Gardner of the Harvard School of Education and Dr. Cecil Mercer of the University of Florida. The 2000 Conference will be in Washington, DC in (November 8 - 11). Our keynote speaker will be Dr. Robert Brooks and the Geschwind Lecture (named for the late Harvard researcher) will be given by Dr. Frank Wood, Wake Forest University

School of Medicine. Future conferences will be held in Albuquerque, New Mexico (2001), Atlanta, Georgia (2002), and San Diego, California (2003). Additionally, IDA recently co-sponsored with the EDA the BDA organized conference on dyslexia in multilingual environments (Manchester, UK – 1999). IDA is planning to sponsor, along with BDA and EDA, a follow-up conference in Washington, DC (June, 2002).

The Publications

IDA publishes many excellent materials, including The Orton Emeritus Series, a group of monographs dealing with the many issues related to dyslexia and our position paper, "Informed Instruction for Reading Success: Foundations for Teacher Preparation." In addition, our magazine, "Perspectives," follows a format of theme issues, covering such issues as assistive technology, tips for parents, and overviews of legal issues. Our "flagship" publication, "Annals of Dyslexia," is one of the premier, peer reviewed journals published in the English language. For information on our publications, please consult our on-line bookstore.

International Dyslexia Association
8600 LaSalle Road
Chester Building, Suite 382
Baltimore, MD 21286-2044, USA

Toll-free (U.S.) (800) ABCD123
Tel: + 410.296.0232
Fax: + 410. 321.5069

Web site: http://www.interdys.org
General e-mail: info@interdys.org

European Dyslexia Association: full speed ahead

As the new President of the European Dyslexia Association, Gyda Skat Nielsen has the task of leading the organisation in its drive to promote dyslexia across Europe. Here she talks about some of the exciting initiatives and changes that are taking place.

In the spring of 1999 the new Board of the European Dyslexia Association started its work. One of the overall objectives of the new Board is to involve each Board Member as much as possible in the work of the Association.

Changes of the structure of the Board of EDA

To run the daily business an Executive Committee has been appointed and a number of Standing Committees have been set up to be responsible for different areas: a Finance Committee, a Marketing and Public Relations Committee, a Membership and Accreditation Committee, a Research Committee and an Internet and Office Committee. Further ad hoc committees will be established when needed. It is possible to invite persons from outside the Board to join the work of the committees.

Close cooperation with the member associations

It is the intention of the Board to create a stronger feeling of belonging to the EDA by involving the member associations as much as possible in our work. For that reason each member association has been asked to appoint a person who will be responsible for contact with the EDA.

To create a better understanding

To overcome certain language barriers which could make the members feel too distant to the EDA, a big effort is being made to have as many of the information materials of the Association as possible translated into the principal languages: German, Spanish and French. Thanks to the new board members from Austria and Switzerland and the German Dyslexia Association (Bundesverband Legasthenie) these efforts have resulted in German translations of EDA News, "Criteria for the Training of Teachers of Dyslexic Students" (1997) and different information materials. The next step will be to encourage the French and Spanish speaking countries to produce translations into their languages in cooperation with the EDA. As the Board of EDA at the moment only has six members it is impossible for the board members alone to do this comprehensive work. Therefore the help and support of the member countries is of major importance.

East-West European Project

One of the aims of the European Dyslexia Association is to provide an international forum for cooperation between its members and others. A good example of this is the "East-West Europe Project" which is planned to take place during 2001, 2002 and 2003. Partners with the EDA will be the Dyslexia Associations in Poland, Hungary and the Czech Republic. During the three years focus will be put on

- Early Recognition
- Education and Training of Children and Adolescents with Dyslexia and
- Adults with Dyslexia: Recognition and Intervention.

One of the main purposes of the Campaign is "to raise awareness of the responsible decision- makers of the magnitude of the problems associated with dyslexia, especially the severe emotional damage which dyslexia can cause and of proven remedial solutions".

There is no doubt that the exchange of experiences between the Eastern and Western European associations will be of invaluable importance for everybody as there is great expertise in both the East and the West for valuable dialogue.

Cyprus Project

Together with the Cyprus Dyslexia Association an interesting project - financially supported by the United Nations (UNOPS) - has started. The Bi-communal Development Program aims at "promoting the peace-building process in Cyprus by encouraging Greek Cypriot and Turkish Cypriot communities to work together in the reparation and implementation of projects in areas of common concern: dyslexia".

IFLA

Another new partner of the EDA is the International Federation of Library Associations and Institutions (IFLA) to whom EDA recently was given a consultative status.

Since the President of EDA was elected a member of the IFLA Section of Libraries Serving Disadvantaged Persons (LSDP), dyslexia has been put on the agenda in the international library world. At the International IFLA Conference in Bangkok 1999 a joint EDA-LSDP Poster Session on dyslexia was presented. The meeting with librarians from all over the world has created important connections in many non-member countries.

At the IFLA International Conference in Boston in 2001, EDA will arrange an Open Session in cooperation with the LSDP and the American International Dyslexia Association (IDA). The theme will be "Raising Awareness of Dyslexia". During the Open Session a new IFLA publication "Guidelines to Library Services to Persons with Dyslexia" by Gyda Skat Nielsen and Birgitta Irvall (Sweden) will be presented and finally a joint EDA-IDA-LSDP booth will present the latest news with information technology for persons with dyslexia and different information materials from the three organizations.

EDA News

The newsletter of the EDA, "EDA News" is published three times a year. Since its new editors, Jennifer and Robin Salter (Great Britain) took over, "EDA News" has undergone different changes and now appears in a modernized format "EDA News" is sent out to all members of the European Dyslexia Association and to a number of individual subscribers. It informs about the work of EDA, interesting things going in the member countries, new books and videos in the field of dyslexia, future conferences and meetings etc. In each issue one of the member associations of the EDA presents itself and its country.

Subscription

Subscription to the EDA Mailing List for individuals remains at £ 5.00 for 3 issues per year

(cheques, eurocheques and overseas money orders accepted). Applications can be send to the EDA Information Center in Brussels.

EDA Information Center

In 1999 the EDA Information Center was formed. Everybody with questions or ideas in relation to dyslexia are welcome to call, fax or e-mail the EDA Information Center.

There is a fast growing number of enquiries from all over the world. Some of these calls are directed on to the national dyslexia associations while others are answered directly by our secretary, Ms. Marty Miller who is working for EDA on a voluntary basis.

For more information please contact
European Dyslexia Association (EDA)
Rue Defacqz 1 1000 Brussels, Belgium
Telephone: 32-2 537 0983
E-mail: eda@compaqnet.be

5th BDA International Conference

DYSLEXIA:
At the dawn of the new century

University of York
18–21 April 2001

Keynote Speakers

Professor Al Galaburda
Dyslexia and the brain

Professor Rod Nicolson
Developmental Dyslexia: into the future

Professor Maggie Snowling
Individual differences and dyslexia

Professor John Stein
Dyslexia and the magnocellular system

Professor Joe Torgesen
Markers for effective intervention

Professor Maryanne Wolf
Dyslexia, fluency and intervention

Please note speakers and programme may be subject to
amendment. Further details and updates will be found
at the conference main website at:
www.bdainternationalconference.org

CReSTeD Explained

CReSTeD - the Council for the Registration of Schools Teaching Dyslexic Pupils - has been operating for over 10 years, and has become recognised as a key reference point when seeking a school with appropriate dyslexia provision. Here Dr Steve Chinn, CReSTeD Chairman, explains the categories.

Category Names and Definitions

Specialist Provision Schools - SP (Formerly Category A)

The school is specifically established to teach pupils with dyslexia and related specific learning difficulties. The curriculum and timetable are designed to meet specific needs in a holistic, co-ordinated manner with a significant number of staff qualified in teaching dyslexic pupils.

Dyslexia Unit - DU (Formerly Category B)

The school has a designated Unit or Centre that provides specialist tuition on a small group or individual basis, according to need. The Unit or Centre is an adequately resourced teaching area under the management of a senior specialist teacher, who co-ordinates the work of other specialist teachers and ensures on-going liaison with all mainstream teachers. This senior specialist teacher will probably have Head of Department status, and will certainly have significant input into the curriculum design and delivery.

Specialist Classes - SC (Formerly Category C)

Schools where dyslexic pupils are taught in separate classes within the school for some lessons, most probably English and mathematics. These are taught by teachers with qualifications in teaching dyslexic pupils. These teachers are deemed responsible for communicating with the pupils' other subject teachers.

Withdrawal System - WS (Formerly Category D)

Schools where dyslexic pupils are withdrawn from appropriately selected lessons for specialist tuition from a teacher qualified in teaching dyslexic pupils. There is on-going communication between mainstream and specialist teachers.

NB 'Qualified' is holding a BDA recognised qualification in the teaching of dyslexic pupils.

Where to obtain the list

For an up-to-date copy of the CReSTeD list please send a stamped addressed envelope (A5) to one of the following places:

British Dyslexia Association
98 London Road, Reading RG1 5AU

The Dyslexia Institute
133 Gresham Road, Staines, Middlesex TW18 2AJ

Christine Manser, CReSTeD Administrator, Greygarth, Littleworth, Winchcombe, Cheltenham GL54 5BT

Tel: 01242 602 689

CReSTeD Criteria

Category	SP	DU	SC	WS
The school is specifically established to teach pupils with dyslexia and related specific learning difficulties.	✔			
Assessment for admission to the school includes EP reports.	✔			
The majority of staff and all English and specialist language teachers are qualified in the teaching of dyslexic children or are undergoing training.	✔			
The school has a designated Unit or Centre that provides specialist tuition on a small group or individual basis.		✔		
The Unit or Centre is adequately resourced, under the management of a senior specialist teacher, who co-ordinates the work of other specialist teachers.		✔		
There is an awareness by other members of staff of the necessity to adjust their teaching to meet the needs of dyslexic pupils and this is evident across the curriculum.		✔		
The Head of Unit or Centre will probably have Head of Department status, and must have an input into curriculum design and delivery.		✔		
The majority of teachers in the Unit or Centre are qualified or are undergoing training in the teaching of dyslexic pupils.		✔		
Dyslexic pupils are taught in separate classes within the school for some lessons, most probably English and mathematics.			✔	
Teachers of these separate classes are responsible for communicating with other subject teachers regarding the dyslexic pupils.			✔	
There is awareness by other members of staff of the needs of dyslexic pupils.			✔	
The majority of specialist teachers are qualified in the teaching of dyslexic pupils or are undergoing training.			✔	✔
There is provision for individual lessons on a withdrawal basis, and these teachers communicate with mainstream teachers regarding the dyslexic pupils.				✔

N.B. 'Qualified' is holding a BDA recognised qualification in the teaching of dyslexic pupils.

PRINCIPAL
Michael Thomson B.Sc, M.Sc, Ph.D,
AFBPsS, FIARLD, C.Psychol.

East Court School
Victoria Parade
Ramsgate
Kent CT11 8ED

Tel. 01843 592077
Fax: 01843 592418

SCHOOL

CReSTeD Category A Approved
British Dyslexia Association Supporting Member

A residential and day school for dyslexic boys and girls aged 8 -13 years.

Aims of East Court

- to help dyslexic children overcome their difficulties and develop their potential.
- to design a structured programme of written language for each child.
- to provide a broad and stimulating education suited to the individual child's needs.
- to make learning fun.

Advantages of East Court

- there is a high level of educational input: all lessons take account of dyslexia.
- there is a high staff to pupil ratio: English and Mathematics are taught in groups of six as well as in smaller groups or one-to-one tutorials.
- all our staff are specialists in helping the dyslexic.
- we are a small, friendly school with a family atmosphere; the whole school is organised to help the dyslexic child in work and leisure.
- the school enables each child to re-enter secondary education no longer dramatically handicapped by being dyslexic.
- we have a wholefood diet and excellent care and pastoral facilities.
- the Principal is an experienced child psychologist as well as a teacher, with many years experience in research, diagnosis and teaching. He is a leading specialists in the field of dyslexia. He has published extensively including the books 'Developmental Dyslexia' (Whurr 1990) and : 'Dyslexia: A teaching handbook' (Whurr 1991) which are standard texts for teacher training.

Further details from: East Court School
Victoria Parade
Ramsgate
Kent CT11 8ED
Tel. 01843 592077   Fax: 01843 592418
E-mail: dyslexia@eastcourtschool.co.uk
Website: www.eastcourtschool.co.uk

Happy and successful dyslexic children at an outstanding, effective school

BDA Accreditation: Dyslexia Qualifications Explained

Lindsay Peer, Education Director and Vice-Chairman of the BDA Accreditation Board writes this short piece on the qualifications that the BDA accredits for those working with dyslexic children and adults.

The Accreditation Board is a prestigious group of professionals which includes representatives from the major teacher training providers in the UK; this includes universities and other training organisations. It is chaired by Professor Bob Burden of Exeter University and supported by the BDA administrative staff.

Specific criteria have been compiled by members of the Board, drawing from their backgrounds in specialist teacher training, educational theory, psychology, research and practice. Criteria exist for the training of teachers, those working in FE/HE and learning support assistants. The qualifications are detailed below.

AMBDA (Associate Membership of the British Dyslexia Association)

This is the highest level of specialist qualification for working with school children. It gives teachers the right to assess and make recommendations for provisions for external public examinations.

ATS (Approved Teacher Status)

As above this is a specialist qualification for working with school children but does not provide the specialist training necessary to qualify teachers to assess for public examination provisions.

AMBDA (FE/HE)

This is the equivalent specialist qualification to AMBDA for working with adults in further and higher education sectors. This includes assessment.

ATS (FE/HE)

This is the equivalent specialist qualification to ATS for working with adults in the further and higher education sectors but does not include assessment for public examinations.

ALSA (Approved Learning Support Assistant)

This qualification gives LSAs the expertise to support dyslexic children in the mainstream classroom under the supervision of the class teacher.

Honorary AMBDA

This is an honorary qualification given to outstanding teacher trainers in the field who began their work before AMBDA was established. There is a minimum requirement of fifteen years dyslexia experience. This is a rare award for which candidates are nominated by two referees.

The qualifications granted by the BDA are recognised by a range of educational bodies including LEAs and the Joint Forum, which is the organisation responsible for examination provisions. All BDA accredited teaching courses are also validated by Higher Education Institutions, which ensures that the highest possible standards are maintained. Courses for Learning Support Assistants are generally overseen by LEAs and have specific elements taught by those holding BDA recognised dyslexia teaching qualifications.

BDA accredited courses are open to teachers who have had a minimum of two years classroom experience, as well as to psychologists and speech and language therapists who have had equivalent professional experience. Eligibility for FE/HE courses requires a minimum of two years experience in the FE/HE sector. Learning Support Assistants, accepted by their LEA for specialist training, may also undertake a BDA accredited course. Entry qualifications for candidates are the responsibility of each individual training institution and not the BDA Accreditation Board.

NEW IN 2000

The BDA TRAINING for TRAINERS Certificate

First awarded in 2000 for those holding either AMBDA or ATS or equivalent, who wished to develop their teacher trainer skills further. This qualification gives them greater knowledge and relevent information to work as tutors in the teacher training world of dyslexia. It is hoped that, within the coming years, all those in the teacher training field will eventually hold this qualification.

AMBDA (Numeracy)

This new diploma is for mainstream teachers working with dyslexic children in the mathematics classroom.

HFBDA (Honorary Fellow of the British Dyslexia Association)

This new award is given to people who have made an outstanding contribution in the field of dyslexia but are not teacher trainers. Candidates need to be nominated by two referees.

We are currently working with the Department for Education and Employment designing a certificate course, which will be for mainstream classroom teachers working in both primary and secondary schools. It is hoped that this will be ready for accreditation in 2001. It will be accredited by Manchester Metropolitan University.

The Accreditation Board also works with educational institutions overseas that are seeking BDA approval. Courses for the teaching of English as an Additional Language to dyslexic students may be approved, to use the training in the assessment procedure and the principle of teaching in ways which are appropriately adapted to local circumstance and needs. This fits with the policy of promoting educational success for dyslexic people around the world.

As you can see there is much happening in the Accreditation world relating to dyslexia. May it go from strength to strength!

BDA WEBSITE
www.bda-dyslexia.org.uk/

Part 2 - About dyslexia

This section tells you about dyslexia, its causes and how to recognise it. It also explains about some of the related specific learning difficulties a dyslexic person may experience.

Part 2 - About dyslexia

What is dyslexia?

*The British Dyslexia Association is often asked wha
by the term 'dyslexia'. Here Lindsay Peer, Educatio
of the BDA, provides us with a description which takes
account of our latest understanding of the strengths and
weaknesses.*

Dyslexia is best described as a combination of abilities and
difficulties which affect the learning process in one or more of
reading, spelling, writing and sometimes numeracy/language.
Accompanying weaknesses may be identified in areas of speed
of processing, short-term memory, sequencing, auditory and/or
visual perception, spoken language and motor skills.

Some children have outstanding creative skills, others have
strong oral skills. Whilst others have no outstanding talents,
they all have strenghts.

Dyslexia occurs despite normal intellectual ability and
conventional teaching. It is independent of socio-economic or
language background.

**It is vital that such children's abilities and
difficulties are identified as early as possible and
that appropriate teaching provision is put in place.**

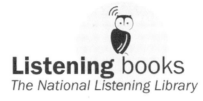
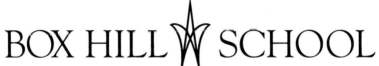

The road to literacy is the road to creativity!

In an attempt to update his analogy of dyslexia, Ian Smythe revisits "the road" and asks if there could be something more than just an analogy!

If we think of the road to literacy as a journey from the town of Langwich to the town of Reading, then dyslexic people have to use back roads

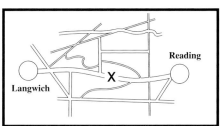

whilst others may use the motorway. Maybe it is not that the road is blocked, but that nobody has shown them the way. So instead they go off in another direction.

The dyslexic person in getting to the destination, finds a different route, explores new worlds, new areas, may boldly go where others fear to tread. He or she can still get to their destination, but they have to take a longer route. It is the role of the teacher to realise that these children can be shown the way, but that they need help to develop strategies to put them on the right track and keep them there.

But now think of all those experiences they may have had along the way. Alas, they are all usually cast aside in the hunt for academic achievement. But is this description, that of finding an alternative route to the destination, just another way of describing creativity? The only difference in this case is that the creativity is not harnessed, but discarded.

Dyslexic individuals can reach their destination if we assist by providing the maps, the knowledge of how to use them, and offer assistance along the way. But let us also harness other ways of seeing.

Recognising dyslexia

There are many persisting factors in dyslexia which can appear from a young age, and still be noticeable when the dyslexic child leaves school. These include:

- obvious "good" and "bad" days, for no apparent reason

- confusion between directional words e.g. up / down; in / out

- difficulty with sequence e.g. coloured bead sequence - later with days of the week, or numbers

- a family history of dyslexia/ reading difficulties

Children who are dyslexic may have a number of the difficulties shown here.

Pre-school

- has persistent jumbled phrases, eg. "cobbler's club" for "toddlers' club"

- use of substitute words, eg. "lampshade" for "lamppost"

- inability to remember the label for known objects eg. table, chair

- difficulty learning nursery rhymes and rhyming words eg. "cat", "mat", "sat"

- finds difficulty in selecting the "odd one out" eg. "cat", "dog", "house", "pig"

- later than expected speech development

Non-language indicators

- may have walked early but did not crawl - was a "bottom shuffler" or "tummy wriggler"

- persistent difficulties in getting dressed efficiently and putting shoes on the correct feet

- enjoys being read to, but shows no interest in letters or words

- is often accused of not listening or paying attention

- excessive tripping, bumping into things and falling over

- difficulty with catching, kicking or throwing a ball, with hopping and/or skipping

- difficulty with clapping a simple rhythm

Primary school age

- has particular difficulty with reading and spelling
- puts letters and figures the wrong way round
- has difficulty remembering tables, alphabet, formulae etc.
- leaves letters out of words or puts them in the wrong order
- still occasionally confuses b and d and words such as no/on
- still needs to use fingers or marks on paper to make simple calculations
- poor concentration
- has problems understanding what s/he has read
- takes longer than average to do written work
- problems processing language at speed

Non-language indicators
- has difficulty with tying shoe laces, tie, dressing
- has difficulty telling left from right, order of days of the week, months of year etc.
- surprises you because in other ways s/he is bright and alert
- has a poor sense of direction and still confuses left and right
- lacks self confidence and has a poor self image

12 or over

As for primary schools, plus:
- still reads inaccurately
- still has difficulties in spelling
- needs to have instructions and telephone numbers repeated
- gets 'tied up' using long words, eg. preliminary, philosophical
- confuses places, times, dates
- has difficulty with planning and writing essays
- has difficulty processing complex language or long series of instructions at speed

Non-language indicators
- has poor confidence and self-esteem
- has areas of strength as well as weakness.

Compiled by Ian Smythe, based on the BDA publication Early Help, Better Future by Jean Augur and extended by Lindsay Peer.

MOON HALL SCHOOL
at BELMONT PREPARATORY SCHOOL

Moon Hall School, Feldemore, Holmbury St. Mary, Dorking, Surrey RH5 6LQ
Telephone: 01306 731464   Fax: 01306 731504
e-mail:enquiries@moonhall.surrey.sch.uk   web address: www.moonhall.surrey.sch.uk
Principal: Mrs J. Lovett, Cert. Ed., AMBDA   Founded: 1985 by Mrs B.E. Baker

....

Status: Independent DfEE registered 936/6551
CReSTeD accredited - Category A

Age range: 7-11 full time
             7-13 part time
Number of Teaching Staff: 15
Type: Mixed

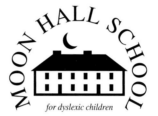
for dyslexic children

Number at Moon Hall:
48 full time
62 part-time
Total Number on site: 260
Weekly Boarding and Day.

Children with Specific Learning Difficulties/Dyslexia benefit from the unique arrangement of a specialist school within a main-stream preparatory school.

Specialist facilities: Full time specialist classes offer a complete curriculum for children aged 7-10, whilst for those over 10, teaching is shared with the Prep. School. Children may attend Moon Hall for specialist tuition in English and Mathematics at all levels. All children benefit from a wide variety of resources available.

General Environment: Moon Hall is in an attractive, homely building in the grounds of Belmont Preparatory School. It shares the facilities of Belmont, including Gym, Dining Room, Library, D&T and I.C.T. facilities, Science Lab, Playing Fields and outdoor Swimming Pool. Belmont School itself is based in an historic Victorian mansion set in 60 acres of wooded grounds. It is mid-way between Dorking and Guildford.

Aims and Philosophy: At Moon Hall we aim to offer sympathetic help to children whose dyslexia affects their ability to learn in a normal classroom. We have helped many highly intelligent dyslexic children to realise their true potential.

Our priority is to restore confidence and to develop a positive attitude to learning. We do this by providing a happy, family atmosphere with support and understanding for each child. However, the demands of any one child are realistically balanced against the needs of the group as a whole.

Children are carefully assessed and given a structured programme appropriate to their needs. The Phono-Graphix reading programme is in use with most of our pupils. This means that they achieve early success on which we can build. We also give them new skills and tools to overcome their difficulties and to build their self esteem. All are taught to touch-type from the age of 7. All benefit from a wide range of specialist reading and spelling computer software. We seek to develop each child's strengths as well as working to overcome their difficulties. Study Skills (including learning techniques, memory techniques, organisation skills etc.) are an important part of our curriculum. Work is based upon the National Curriculum and Common Entrance Examination where appropriate. Our eventual aim is to return any child who is able, to a mainstream class - usually Belmont - with ongoing support.

Home/School Links: Moon Hall School has close links with all parents. Regular written reports are issued - including syllabus reports. There are Parents' Evenings and regular talks about our work. A thriving and well-supported PTA exists and this organises social functions and fund raising events. Boarding at Belmont is on a weekly basis and children are therefore free for a full family weekend from Fridays at 4.30 p.m.

Staff qualifications: All staff are fully qualified in their own field and each member of the English Staff has a Diploma in the Assessment and Teaching of Children with Specific Learning Difficulties/Dyslexia. Staff regularly attend National Conferences etc. and we are involved in several areas of important research. Most staff now have an additional Phono-Graphix qualification.

Checklist for dyslexic adults

There are many ways in which checklists for dyslexic adults may be used. Whilst it will not provide enough information for a diagnostic assessment it can be very useful in providing a better self-understanding and be a pointer towards future assessment needs. Here, Ian Smythe and John Everatt (University of Surrey) explain their work.

In an attempt to overcome the difficulties of previous checklists, (eg the use of just 'Yes' and 'No' as possible answers), we have, over the last few years, been piloting and testing a new checklist for dyslexic adults which is set out here for the first time. The results are based on extensive questioning in many contexts, and not just within the traditional area of higher education. The results have provided a valuable insight into the diversity of difficulties, and is a clear reminder that every individual is different and should be treated and assessed as such. However, it is also interesting to note that a number of questions, the answers to which are said to be characteric of dyslexic adults, are commonly found also in the answers of non-dyslexics.

On the following two pages are the questions that were found to be most predictive of dyslexia (as measured by prior diagnosis). The full set of questions provides more information on the diversity of difficulties. (The full questionnaire is available at http://web.ukonline.co.uk/wdnf/adultcheck.html). In order to provide what we consider to be the most informative checklist, we have allowed answers from 'Rarely' (score 1) to 'Most of the time' (score 4) in Part 1, or Easy (score 1) to Difficult (score 4) in Part 2. Alongside each line you can keep a tally of what you score, and in the end find a total.

The Checklist (Part 1)

*For each question circle the box which is closest to your response from **Rarely** to **Most of the time**. For example, if you frequently have trouble filling in forms, put a circle around 3 (the number in the 'Frequently' column), and write the number again under the 'Total' column.*

	Rarely	Occasionally	Frequently	Most of the time	Total
1. Do you confuse visually similar words when reading (e.g. tan, ton)?	3	6	9	12	
2. Do you lose your place or miss out lines when reading?	2	4	6	8	
3. Do you confuse the names of objects (e.g. table for chair)?	1	2	3	4	
4. Do you have trouble telling left from right?	1	2	3	4	
5. Is map reading or finding your way to a strange place confusing?	1	2	3	4	
6. Do you re-read paragraphs to understand them?	1	2	3	4	
7. Do you get confused when given several instructions at once?	1	2	3	4	
8. Do you make mistakes when taking down telephone messages?	1	2	3	4	
9. Do you find it difficult to find the right word to say?	1	2	3	4	

Total so far [ ]

The Checklist (Part 2)

*For each question circle the box which is closest to your response from **Easy** to **Very difficult**.
For example, if you find sounding out words difficult, put a circle around 3 (the number in the 'Difficult' column), and write the number again under the 'Total' column.*

	Easy	Challenging	Difficult	Very difficult	Total
Total from Part 1 (questions 1-9)					
10. How easy do you find it to sound out words? (E.g. el-e-phant)	3	6	9	12	
11. When writing do you find it difficult to organise thoughts on paper?	2	4	6	8	
12. Did you learn your multiplication tables easily?	2	4	6	8	
13. How easy is it for you to learn to write a foreign language?	1	2	3	4	
14. How easy do you find it to recite the alphabet?	1	2	3	4	
15. How easy is it to think of unusual (creative) solutions to problems?	1	2	3	4	
16. How hard do you find it to read aloud?	1	2	3	4	

Total score

Results from the adult test – What it all means

It is important to remember that this does not constitute an assessment of one's difficulties. It is just an indication of some of the areas in which you, or the person you are assessing, may have difficulties. It is important to stress that only through an extensive assessment carried out by those who have a real understanding of the potential difficulties can a full understanding of the difficulties be reached. However, this questionnaire may provide a better awareness of the nature of the difficulties. If you use this questionnaire it should be for personal interest and should not as yet be used to decide whether to seek further support.

Whilst we do stress that this is not a diagnostic tool, we can state that our research suggests the following:

Score less than 45 – probably non-dyslexic

Research result: no individual who was diagnosed as dyslexic through a full assessment was found to have scored less than 42, and therefore it is unlikely that if you score under 42, you will be dyslexic.

Score 45-60 – showing signs consistent with mild dyslexia

Research result: most of those who were in this category showed signs of being at least moderately dyslexic. However, a number of persons not diagnosed as dyslexic (though they could just be unrecognised and undiagnosed) also fell in this category.

Score greater than 60 – signs consistent with moderate or severe dyslexia

Research result: all those who recorded score of more than 60 were diagnosed as moderately or severely dyslexic. Therefore we would suggest that a score greater than 60 suggest moderately or severely dyslexic.

Please note that this should not be regarded as an assessment of one's difficulties. But if you feel that a dyslexia type problem may exist, further advice should be sought. Your local College of Further Education or University Learning Support team may be able to advise if you are studying or considering further study.

Your local dyslexia association may also be able to help. See the blue pages for a full listing.

If you have any further problems please telephone the BDA Helpline 0118 966 8271.

For further details about this research, please contact Ian Smythe: Email ian.smythe@ukonline.co.uk

ADULT DYSLEXIA & SKILLS DEVELOPMENT CENTRE

The aims of the Centre are to help adult dyslexics achieve their full potential, and younger dyslexics to become successful adults through individual counselling training and teaching.

Each person attending the Centre will be provided with an individual programme designed to meet their particular needs.

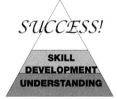

SUCCESS!

SKILL
DEVELOPMENT
UNDERSTANDING

"Success through Understanding and Skills Development"

For further information please contact us at
5 Tavistock Place, London WC1H 9SN
Telephone: 020 7388 8744   Fax: 020 7388 8744
Email: dyslexia@adsdc.freeserve.co.uk

THE OLD RECTORY SCHOOL
Brettenham, Ipswich, Suffolk.

Co-educational Dyslexia School
Ages 7-13
Number of Pupils: Boys 39, Girls 9. Number of Boarders: 37
Fees: on application

THE OLD RECTORY IS A SPECIALIST SCHOOL FOR CHILDREN who are suffering from specific learning difficulties - commonly called Dyslexia.

The school is accredited by the National Registration Council (CReSTeD) and is a Supporting Corporate Member of the BRITISH DYSLEXIA ASSOCIATION.

The aim of the Old Rectory is to help children realise their true potential within a family environment. In their past schooling they may well have been misunderstood and their problems blamed on laziness or stupidity. Constant failure may well have resulted in the child suffering from a severe lack of confidence which will only be corrected in a sympathetic and understanding environment. It is for this reason that the Old Rectory was established. Children enjoy the comfort, security and care of a family atmosphere as well as receiving specialist and individual remedial help.

Although the emphasis is on the acquisition of literacy and numeracy skills, all children follow the National Curriculum.

Depending on the severity of their difficulties and on their progress, children remain at the Old Rectory for a **minimum of one year and a maximum of two years.** The Headteacher believes that it is her mutual responsibility with parents, to find suitable placement in other schools when children leave.

The Old Rectory is set in 5 acres of landscaped grounds at the edge of a peaceful Suffolk village adjacent to the church and enjoys uninterrupted country views in all directions.

Details from: The Secretary
The Old Rectory School, Brettenham, Ipswich, Suffolk IP7 7QR
Tel: 01449 736404   Fax: 01449 737881
Headteacher: Ann Furlong MA. Cert Ed, Dip Sp Needs Ed, Dip SpLD

Research - into the new millennium

As Chair of the 5th International Dyslexia Conference, Professor Rod Nicolson looks forward to an exciting event, and reviews what directions current reserach is taking. He highlights some of the work that is currently going on, and which can be heard at the conference.

Over the years, the BDA International Conferences have developed an outstanding reputation for providing a stimulating, sociable and state of the art survey of dyslexia research and practice. We expect 'Dyslexia: At the Dawn of the New Century' to be even more successful.

The conference takes place from Wednesday 18th to Saturday 21st of April 2001 at the University of York. There has been a record entry of high quality submissions, with nearly 300 accepted as workshops, papers or posters. We have grouped them into broad themes -

Biological bases

Cognitive processes

Theory and Good Practice for 0-5 years,

Theory and Good Practice for 5-11 years,

Theory and Good Practice for 11-18 years

Dyslexia in Adulthood

Screening and diagnosis

Multilingual and international perspectives

Social and emotional aspects

Dyslexia and other learning disabilities.

I start the keynote lectures by highlighting the outstanding progress - theoretical and applied - that has been made in the past decade. I then pose six questions for dyslexia research:

1) What are the potential underlying causes of dyslexia?

2) How can we identify each 'subtype'?

3) How should we support each 'subtype'?

4) What are the targets for support at different ages?

5) What is the relationship between dyslexia and other learning disabilities?

6) How can we co-ordinate research and practice to achieve our dyslexia objectives?

In the course of the conference we will all hear much that will bear on these issues. Other keynote speakers include:

Maryanne Wolf, who will be talking about her influential theory (with Pat Bowers) - the 'double deficit' theory of dyslexia - which suggests that dyslexic children suffer from the twin problems of poor phonological processing and also slow speed of processing.

Joe Torgesen describes the systematic US analyses of the 'optimal' rate of growth in literacy for dyslexic children following successful interventions, and continues with an analysis of why some interventions are more effective than others.

Maggie Snowling addresses the further important issue that not all dyslexic children are the same, and presents an analysis of individual differences in responses to intervention.

John Stein then presents his challenging theory that most problems of dyslexic children stem directly or indirectly from sensory processing problems, attributable in turn to abnormal magnocellular pathways.

Al Galaburda, one of the pioneers of brain research in

dyslexia, will present fascinating insights from 20 years of research on the brain.

In addition to the keynotes there is lots for everyone. I expect highlights to include the infancy symposium, in which Heikki Lyytinnen and his collaborators present the fascinating results of the Finnish national longitudinal study in which 200 children with dyslexic families were followed through from birth to (so far) 6 years; their cognitive performance and sensory processing capabilities were examined minutely. Results to date suggest that there may well be significant differences in scalp-recorded EEG responses to speech-based sounds even immediately after birth. We have a particularly strong genetics symposium, with most of the key international groups represented, which describes how the development of new genotyping technology and statistical methodology has allowed researchers to begin to identify locations of genetic factors that may be implicated in dyslexia, though there is still considerable debate in the area.

The vision symposium, chaired by Piers Cornelissen, investigates the likely role of visual abnormalities on reading problems, with particular analysis of the issue of reduced sensitivity to visual motion. The early support symposium presents powerful data on the importance of a 'stitch in time', demonstrating that if appropriate support is given at nursery age, many children at risk of dyslexia will in fact learn to read reasonably normally.

There are also equally encouraging and important sessions and symposia in the themes on Theory and Good Practice 5-11 years and 11-18 years. The 'English as an Additional Language' symposium, chaired by Tony Cline, continues with the outstanding research presented at the 1999 BDA Multilingual Conference in Manchester. Continuing further important theoretical themes from that conference, there are several important talks on multilingual issues in dyslexia - both

from the point of view of languages other than English and for children learning several languages.

Adults are also well represented with symposia on adults and on dyslexia in higher education. We are fortunate to have a strong international presence, and there should be a number of fascinating presentations, including Priscilla Vail talking on dyslexia and giftedness.

There are two very strong poster sessions. I actually find these sessions even more valuable than the talks, in that we get the opportunity to have real conversations about the key issues, rather than just abbreviated questions and answers.

In parallel with the paper and poster sessions, but scheduled to avoid clashes of like topics, we have 20 workshops, mostly covering good practice and teaching, and promising outstanding opportunities to enjoy 'hands on' interactions.

On the Saturday, following the keynote we include some more controversial contributions, including a symposium on alternative treatments of dyslexia and a symposium on strengths of dyslexic people. We follow the morning session with three parallel 'Round Table' sessions - 'Causal Theories of Dyslexia', 'Identification and Support' and 'Policy' respectively, in which a selected panel sits round the table, each presents a brief overview, and the audience participates, with the intention of developing shared visions of future progress. The conference culminates with a final large round table session where all three groups pool their thoughts in the main auditorium, followed by Concluding Comments.

My aim as Conference Chair has been to encourage a broad view of dyslexia, nationally and internationally, considering both 'pure' and 'applied' theoretical research, and how the research findings feed into recommendations on good practice. I take the view that differences in approach are likely to lead to different emphases and different findings. These are healthy indicators of an emerging discipline. If we listen carefully to the practitioners as well as the theorists we are likely to make very significant progress not only in the scientific understanding of dyslexia but also in the support for children and adults with dyslexia .

See page 56 for the list of Keynote Speakers. Further details and updates will be found at the conference main website at:

www.bdainternationalconference.org

DYSLEXIA:
At the dawn of the new century
18−21 April 2001

Directory

This section contains details of local dyslexia associations and other organisations where you can get help and support.

This information is as correct as possible at the time of printing. Contact details may subsequently change. If you have any problems, please check with BDA Helpline Tel: 0118 966 8271 E-mail: info@dyslexiahelp-bda.demon.co.uk Web: http://www.bda-dyslexia.org.uk/

Local dyslexia association helplines in England, Northern Ireland and Wales

BDA Local Area - Central 1

Anglesey
Blaenau Gwent
Bridgend
Caerphilly
Cardiff
Cardiganshire
Carmarthenshire
Conwy
Denbighshire
Flintshire
Glamorgan, Vale of

Gwynedd
Merthyr Tydfil
Monmouthshire
Neath and Port Talbot
Newport
Pembrokeshire
Powys
Rhonda Cynon Taff
Swansea
Torfaen
Wrexham

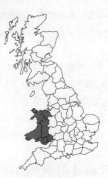

Local Dyslexia Associations and their Helplines

Please note that most helplines are answered by volunteers at home. Where no adult helpliner is listed, general helpliners take adult enquiries. If you have problems with any of these numbers, please check with BDA Helpline, Tel: 0118 966 8271 E-mail: info@dyslexiahelp-bda.demon.co.uk or see Web: http://www.bda-dyslexia.org.uk/

Gwent DA	01633 267 268	
Gwynedd DA	01286 673 122	LL23-90, SY
Gwynedd DA	01248 810 203	LL23-90, SY
NE Wales DA	01691 772 028	
NE Wales DA	01352 770 033	
West Wales DA	0402 665 799	Postcodes Swansea and West Wales
	www.swansea.gov.uk/wwda	

BDA Local Area - Central 2

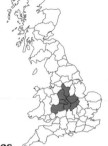

Birmingham
Coventry
Dudley
Herefordshire
Leicester, City of
Leicestershire
Northamptonshire
Rutland

Sandwell
Solihull
Staffordshire
Stoke on Trent, City of
Walsall
Warwickshire
Wolverhampton
Worcester

Local Dyslexia Associations and their Helplines

Please note that most helplines are answered by volunteers at home. Where no adult helpliner is listed, general helpliners take adult enquiries. Birmingham Adult DG covers many West Midlands areas. If you have problems with any of these numbers, please check with BDA Helpline, Tel: 0118 966 8271
E-mail: info@dyslexiahelp-bda.demon.co.uk or see Web: http://www.bda-dyslexia.org.uk/

Birmingham DA	0121 643 3737	
Birmingham Adult DG	07071 710 071	Birmingham postcodes
		Ansafone:evening response
Dudley DA	01902 885 701	DY postcodes
	kimhatton@allcomm.co.uk	
Hereford & Worcester DA	01905 723 168	Postcodes HR, WR, DY, B
	sj_jones@hwda.demon.co.uk	
	www.hwda.demon.co.uk	
Hereford & Worcester DA	01905 840 979	Postcodes HR, WR, DY, B
Hereford & Worcester DA	01905 840 979	Adults.
Leicestershire DA	0455 633 673	Hinckley
	NFlintham@aol.com	
Leicestershire DA	01664 851 890	Melton Mowbray
Leicestershire DA	0116 241 2480	LE postcodes
Leicestershire DA	0116 271 6354	LE postcodes
Leicestershire DA	0116 212 7420	Market Harborough
Leicestershire DA	0116 210 7588	Adults. Evenings
Leicestershire DA	01509 414 205	Loughborough
Northamptonshire DA	01604 493 103	9am-8pm or ansafone.
	www.northantsda.freeserve.co.uk/	
Rugby & District DA	024 7627 9799	W/day 4-8pm. W/end 10-6
Rutland DA	01664 454 185	Adults. Evenings.
Rutland DA	01780 720 742	Evenings
	kay_jaques@email.msn.com	
DA for Walsall Now (DAWN)	01922 867 764	Postcodes WS, WV
	dawndyslexia@yahoo.com	
North Warwickshire DA	024 7632 0169	Postcodes CV1-13,
	lesleyhilldysl@beeb.net	B46,76,78,79.
South Warwickshire DA	01386 792 252	
South Warwickshire DA	01789 773 758	

BDA Local Area - Central 3

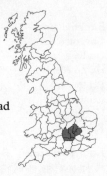

Bedfordshire	Oxfordshire
Bracknell	Reading
Buckinghamshire	Slough
Hertfordshire	West Berkshire
Luton	Windsor and Maidenhead
Milton Keynes	Wokingham

Local Dyslexia Associations and their Helplines

Please note that most helplines are answered by volunteers at home. Where no adult helpliner is listed, general helpliners take adult enquiries. If you have problems with any of these numbers, please check with BDA Helpline, Tel: 0118 966 8271
E-mail: info@dyslexiahelp-bda.demon.co.uk or see Web: http://www.bda-dyslexia.org.uk/

Bedford DA	01234 881 345	MK 40-45, SG17-19
South Bedfordshire DA	01582 752 444	Also Luton. Ansafone
West Berkshire DA	01635 298 864	RG7-20
South Buckinghamshire DA	01494 534 872	HP5-16, SL1,2,7-9.
Hertfordshire DA	01923 265 031	AL, CM, HP, SG, WD
Oxfordshire DA	01865 873 547	
Oxfordshire DA	01865 558 273	
Reading DA	0118 978 3363	Wokingham
Reading DA	0118 984 2549	Reading. Before 9pm.
		RG1, 2, 4-8, 10, 30, 31, 40, 41
DA of Windsor & Maidenhead	01344 455 514	Bracknell. Evenings
Slough & Bracknell		
DA of Windsor & Maidenhead	01628 676 055	Windsor and Maidenhead
Slough & Bracknell		Evenings
DA of Windsor & Maidenhead	01753 522 020	Slough. Evenings
Slough & Bracknell		

BDA Local Area - Central 4

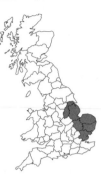

Cambridgeshire
Derby, City of
Derbyshire
Essex
Lincolnshire
Norfolk
North East Lincolnshire

North Lincolnshire
Nottingham, City of
Nottinghamshire
Peterborough
Southend
Suffolk
Thurrock

Local Dyslexia Associations and their Helplines

Please note that most helplines are answered by volunteers at home. Where no adult helpliner is listed, general helpliners take adult enquiries. If you have problems with any of these numbers, please check with BDA Helpline, Tel: 0118 966 8271 E-mail: info@dyslexiahelp-bda.demon.co.uk or see Web: http://www.bda-dyslexia.org.uk/

Cambridge DA	01223 834 615	
Nottinghamshire DA	0115 958 8400	Also Derby, Lincs.
	Helpline@theNDA.fsnet.co.uk	
	www.nottsdyslexia.com	
Peterborough & District DA	01733 211 022	
	paulby@globalnet.co.uk	
Suffolk DA	01473 310 236	
Suffolk DA	01284 753 047	
Central Suffolk & District DA	01449 614 747	
Waveney Valley DA	01379 668 430	Norfolk
	BRAWhiting@aol.com	
Waveney Valley DA	01603 618 949	Norfolk
	WVDyslexia@aol.com	

BDA Local Area - North 1

Cumbria
Darlington
Durham
Gasteshead
Hartlepool
Middlesborough
Newcastle upon Tyne

North Tyneside
Northern Ireland
Northumberland
Redcar & Cleveland
South Tyneside
Stockton on Tees
Sunderland

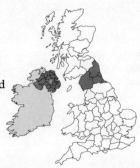

Local Dyslexia Associations and their Helplines

Please note that most helplines are answered by volunteers at home. Where no adult helpliner is listed, general helpliners take adult enquiries. If you have problems with any of these numbers, please check with BDA Helpline, Tel: 0118 966 8271
E-mail: info@dyslexiahelp-bda.demon.co.uk or see Web: http://www.bda-dyslexia.org.uk/

North Cumbria DA	01768 361 867	Postcodes CA
South Cumbria DA	01229 828 120	Postcodes LA9, 11-15,
	PhylPDysl@aol.com	18, 19, 23
South Cumbria DA	01539 738 376	Postcodes LA9, 11-15,
		18, 19, 23
West Cumbria DA	07000 782 171	CA13-28
	Christine.dyslexia@talk21.com	
Darlington & D DSG	01325 387 700	Mon-Thur 8.30am-8.45pm
		Friday 8.30am-5.00pm
Darlington & D DSG	01325 462 523	Durham
	carol@saxbys.freeserve.co.uk	
Hartlepool DA	01429 276 064	Postcodes TS24-27
	Hartlepooldyslexia@care4free.net	
Northern Ireland DA	028 9066 0111	
	nida@dnet.co.uk	
Central Tyneside DA	0191 488 0819	

Another useful contact:
DA of Ireland

00 1 679 0276
acld@iol.ie
www.acld-dyslexia.com

BDA Local Area - North 2

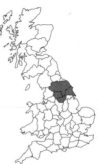

Barnsley
Bradford
Calderdale
Doncaster
East Riding of Yorkshire
Hull/Kingston Upon Hull
Kirklees

Leeds
North Yorkshire
Rotherham
Sheffield
Wakefield
York, City of

Local Dyslexia Associations and their Helplines

Please note that most helplines are answered by volunteers at home. Where no adult helpliner is listed, general helpliners take adult enquiries. If you have problems with any of these numbers, please check with BDA Helpline, Tel: 0118 966 8271
E-mail: info@dyslexiahelp-bda.demon.co.uk or see Web: http://www.bda-dyslexia.org.uk/

Calderdale DA	01422 884 206	HD6, HX1-7, OL14.
	michaelairey@northvale.sagehost.co.uk	
Doncaster DA	01302 816 070	Resource Centre.
		Mon-Fri, 9.30-5.30
Kirklees DA	01924 407 920	Daytime only. BD19,HD1-8,
		WF12-15,17 & parts of others.
Kirklees DA	01924 491 487	Evenings only. BD19,HD1-8,
		WF12-15,17 & parts of others.
Leeds & Bradford DA	01757 288 889	Postcodes BD, LS.
Leeds & Bradford DA	01274 771 153	Postcodes BD, LS.
	jane@labda.org.uk	Postcodes BD, LS. Also adults.
	www.labda.org.uk	9.30am-9.30pm every day
Leeds & Bradford DA	0113 266 1947	Postcodes BD, LS.
Sheffield & District DA	01246 865 318	

BDA Local Area - North 3

Blackburn
Blackpool
Bolton
Bury
Lancashire
Manchester

Oldham
Rochdale
Salford
Sefton
Wigan

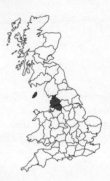

Local Dyslexia Associations and their Helplines

Please note that most helplines are answered by volunteers at home. Where no adult helpliner is listed, general helpliners take adult enquiries. If you have problems with any of these numbers, please check with BDA Helpline, Tel: 0118 966 8271
E-mail: info@dyslexiahelp-bda.demon.co.uk or see Web: http://www.bda-dyslexia.org.uk/

Bolton & District DA	01204 848 722	9am-4pm or ansafone
Lancaster & District DA	01524 400 395	LA1-6.
Oldham DA	01706 881 792	
Preston & District DA	01772 617 248	Evenings & weekends
		PR2-7, FY4, 6, 8, BB3
Preston & District DA	01253 738 414	Daytime & evenings
		PR2 7, FY4, 6, 8, BB3
Preston & District DA	01772 863 580	Any time
		PR2-7, FY4, 6, 8, BB3
Salford DA	0161 775 3071	Postcodes M5-7, 27, 28,
		29, 30, 38, 44
Southport & District DA	01704 541 511	PR8,9, L10, L20-23,
		L29-31, L37-40, WN8
Wigan & District DA	01942 202 255	8-10pm or ansafone
	WaDDA1111@aol.com	Mon-Fri

Another useful contact:
Manx DA

01624 843 392
mwca@pridham21.freeserve.co.uk

BDA Local Area - North 4

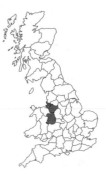

Cheshire
Halton
Knowsley
Liverpool
Shropshire
St Helens

Stockport
Tameside
Telford & Wrekin
Trafford
Warrington
Wirral

Local Dyslexia Associations and their Helplines

Please note that most helplines are answered by volunteers at home. Where no adult helpliner is listed, general helpliners take adult enquiries. If you have problems with any of these numbers, please check with BDA Helpline, Tel: 0118 966 8271
E-mail: info@dyslexiahelp-bda.demon.co.uk or see Web: http://www.bda-dyslexia.org.uk/

Cheshire DA	01829 741 710	Or Ansafone
	c.da@virgin.net	
	http://freespace.virgin.net/jim.middleton	
Cheshire DA	01829 741 710	Or Ansafone
	c-armitage@s-cheshire.ac.uk Adults	
Liverpool DA	0151 724 5758	Ansafone. L1-8,11-19, 24,25,27, parts of L9,10.
Shropshire DA	01743 231 205	
Shropshire DA	01743 340 878	
St Helens DA	01744 612 276	Helpline rota. L34,35,
	StHelensDA@box42.com	WA2,8-12, WN4,5.
Stockport DA	0161 431 3641	SK postcodes
Stockport DA	0161 440 0842	SK postcodes
Trafford DA	0161 973 6911	Postcodes M4, 16, 17, 30-33,41,42,90, WA14,15
DA (Wirral)	0151 652 6005	Adults
	Blease@kingsmead.netideas.co.uk	
		Postcodes CH45-66
DA (Wirral)	0151 653 4040	Tues 6-8, Fri 10-12, Sat 2-4
	neil.f@which.net	Termtime or ansafone

BDA Local Area - South 1

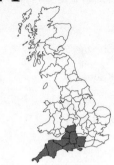

Bath and NE Somerset	North Somerset
Bournemouth	Plymouth
Bristol, City of	Poole
Channel Islands	Portsmouth, City of
Cornwall	Somerset
Devon	South Gloucestershire
Dorset	Southampton
Gloucestershire	Swindon
Hampshire	Torbay
Isle of Wight	Wiltshire

Local Dyslexia Associations and their Helplines

Please note that most helplines are answered by volunteers at home. Where no adult helpliner is listed, general helpliners take adult enquiries. If you have problems with any of these numbers, please check with BDA Helpline, Tel: 0118 966 8271 E-mail: info@dyslexiahelp-bda.demon.co.uk or see Web: http://www.bda-dyslexia.org.uk/

Bristol DA	0117 904 3452	Ansafone gives info & enquirers are contacted
Cornwall DA	01872 274 827	Rota. All TR, some PL postcodes
Devon DA	01803 712 763 c.pett@tesco.net	Also adults
Devon DA	01404 812 980	
Devon DA	01392 468 276	Also adults
Dorset DA	01202 698 617 Tonyhamltn@aol.com	Postcodes DT, BH, SP
Gloucestershire DA	01242 238 080	GL7 postcodes. Adults.
Gloucestershire DA	01242 222 328	GL postcodes. Ansafone
Gloucestershire South DA	01452 615 512	GL21-45. 24hr helpline
Hampshire DA	023 8033 3345	Mon&Thur 10-12noon. Tues10-2.30pm. SO, RG, PO, GU
Isle of Wight DA	01983 565 024	Evenings
Jersey DA	01534 741 841	
Somerset DA	01278 732 671	
DA for N Somerset	01934 625 298 cpcjn@breathemail.net	
DA for N Somerset	01934 645 728 robert@cabot-house.freeserve.co.uk	Also Adults.
Wiltshire DA	01249 811 971 Nigel.Pugh@tesco.net	

BDA Local Area - South 2

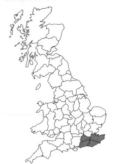

Brighton & Hove
East Sussex
Kent
Medway
Surrey
West Sussex

Local Dyslexia Associations and their Helplines

Please note that most helplines are answered by volunteers at home. Where no adult helpliner is listed, general helpliners take adult enquiries. If you have problems with any of these numbers, please check with BDA Helpline, Tel: 0118 966 8271
E-mail: info@dyslexiahelp-bda.demon.co.uk or see Web: http://www.bda-dyslexia.org.uk/

Kent Central DA	01622 755 515	ME14-20.
Kent Central DA	01435 872 856	Evenings, weekends
	SuMFallon@aol.com	
	http://members.tripod.co.uk/kcda	
South Kent DA	01233 850 273	Postcodes CT, ME13, TN17,18,21,23-30
South Kent DA	01233 335 496	Evens & School holidays Postcodes CT, ME13, TN17,18,21,23-30
Kent West DA	01959 561 978	Helpline. TN1-18, ME19, DA3,13
Kent West DA	01732 458 857	Information Line. TN1-18, ME19, DA3,13
Medway DA	01634 371 802	Adults
Medway DA	01634 848 232	Postcodes ME1-13, DA1-4
	barry@wjames.freeserve.co.uk	
South East Surrey DA	01883 712 224	RH1-9, CR3, CR6, SM7,
	jan-warne@hotmail.com	KT18, KT20
West Surrey DAA	01252 338 005	GU postcodes, KT11,12,22
East Sussex DA	01424 211 897	Also part Brighton & Hove
East Sussex DA	01273 584 041	Also part Brighton & Hove
East Sussex DA	01323 896 542	Adults, B&H, W Sx.
	nicky@woodward3040.freeserve.co.uk	
West Sussex DA	01903 532 952	Weekdays 2-4pm Also part Brighton & Hove
West Sussex DA	01428 741 013	Weekdays 5-8pm Also part Brighton & Hove
West Sussex DA	01903 714 208	4-6pm Also part Brighton & Hove

BDA Local Area - South 3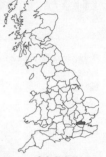

Greater London (North)

Local Dyslexia Associations and their Helplines

Please note that most helplines are answered by volunteers at home. Where no adult helpliner is listed, general helpliners take adult enquiries. London Adult SG covers adult enquiries from most of the London Dyslexia Support Groups. If you have problems with any of these numbers, please check with BDA Helpline, Tel: 0118 966 8271
E-mail: info@dyslexiahelp-bda.demon.co.uk or see Web: http://www.bda-dyslexia.org.uk/

Barking & Dagenham DA	01708 501 945	Evenings. Also Havering.
Barnet DA	020 8958 7452	Ansafone
	iceldevp@btinternet.com	
Brent DSG (London DA)	020 8969 6038	Weekday evenings after 7pm
	I.J.Schiemann@lse.ac.uk	
Ealing DA	020 8995 7092	Most times. Also Hounslow. W3,5,7,13,UB1,2,6
Ealing DA	020 8995 7092	Adults. After sunset. Also Hounslow
Enfield & District DA	020 8367 2490	EN1-3,4(part),N9,11,13,14,18,21
	pjking@fivekings.freeserve.co.uk	
Enfield & District DA	020 8292 5671	Daytime, termtime EN1-3,4(part),N9,11,13,14,18,21
Hackney DSG (London DA)	020 8806 6965	
Haringey DSG (London DA)	020 8348 4292	Monday 5-7pm. N4,6,8-11,15,16,17,22
Haringey DSG (London DA)	020 8444 9857	Thursday 7-9pm. N4,6,8-11,15,16,17,22
Harrow SPELD	020 8868 4523	HA0-9 evenings only
Hillingdon DA	01895 673 288	Postcodes HA4-6, UB
	hdahelpline@yahoo.co.uk	
	http://members.tripod.co.uk/Hillda/	
Hillingdon DA	01895 657 530	Postcodes HA4-6, UB
Islington (London DA)	020 7609 7515	N1,4,5,7,19,EC1,WC1
London DA	020 7407 0900	Mon-Fri 10am-12, 2-4pm Camden, City, Hammersmith & Fulham, Kensington & Chelsea, Lambeth, Newham, Southwark, Westminster
London Adult SG (London DA)	020 8870 1407	Ansafone. Adults
Redbridge DSG (London DA)	020 8554 5889	Mon-Fri. 10am-3pm.
Redbridge DSG (London DA)	020 8505 5984	Mon-Fri. 8-10pm.
Tower Hamlets DSG (London DA)	020 8471 9207	10-2.30pm; after 6pm
Tower Hamlets DSG (London DA)	020 8983 1397	Evenings only
Waltham Forest DA	020 8989 4629	Postcodes E4,10,11,17

BDA Local Area - South 4

Greater London (South)

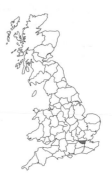

Local Dyslexia Associations and their Helplines

Please note that most helplines are answered by volunteers at home. Where no adult helpliner is listed, general helpliners take adult enquiries. London Adult SG covers adult enquiries from most of the London Dyslexia Support Groups. If you have problems with any of these numbers, please check with BDA Helpline, Tel: 0118 966 8271
E-mail: info@dyslexiahelp-bda.demon.co.uk or see Web: http://www.bda-dyslexia.org.uk/

Croydon DA	020 8656 7269	CR0-8
Croydon DA	020 8657 3612	CR0-8
Croydon DA	020 8409 0127	Evenings only. CR0-8
North Kent DA	020 8319 3662	Bexley, Bromley, Greenwich. Adults only.
North Kent DA	020 8467 9264 lindy.springett@virgin.net www.nkda.freeserve.co.uk	Bexley, Bromley, Greenwich
North Kent DA	07000 50 50 55	Bexley, Bromley, Greenwich. Rota.
Kingston DA	0961 375 561	KT1-24
Lewisham ADS (N Kent DA)	020 8857 7369	Tues, Wed 7-8.30pm. Or ansafone
Merton & SW London DA	020 8682 0773	After 6pm. Also Wandsworth.
Merton & SW London DA	020 8946 0469	After 6pm. Also Wandsworth.
Merton & SW London DA	020 8947 1674	Adults. Also Wandsworth.
Merton & SW London DA	020 8241 6118	After 6pm. Also Wandsworth.
Richmond DA	020 8332 2881	Tues am. Sun evenings. Postcode SW,TW, some KT
Richmond DA	020 8878 2434	Mon am, Wed, Thurs 6-9pm
Sutton DA	020 8668 4209 Helpline@suttondyslexia.org.uk www.suttondyslexia.org.uk	Postcodes SM1-7

Scottish Dyslexia Association Helpline Numbers

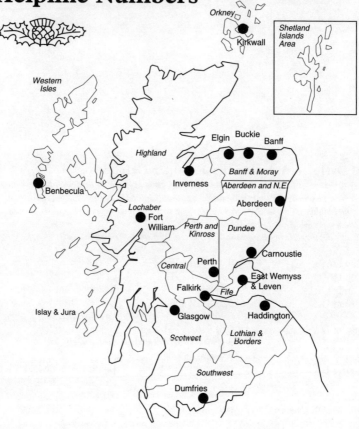

The Scottish Dyslexia Association has an extensive network of local helplines and support, as indicated in the map above. For details on how to contact them, please call our Head Office.

Scottish Dyslexia Association
Stirling Business Centre, Wellgreen Place, Stirling FK8 2DZ
Telephone: 01786 446650   Fax: 01786 471235
E-mail: dyslexia.scotland@dial.pipex.com
Web: www.dyslexia.scotland.dial.pipex.com

Supporting Corporate Members of the BDA

BDA Supporting Corporate Members support BDA's aims and objectives and agree to abide by its Membership Code.

These establishments offer one or more of the following services: A= Assessment, B= Books and/or software, C= Consultancy, FE= Further Education, HE= Higher Education, M= Mainstream School, R= Research, S= Specialist School, TC= Teaching Centre, TTC= Teacher Training courses.

Supporting Corporate Members will be able to give you further information about their qualifications, fees, facilities and age ranges.

Some schools on this list are CReSTeD members (see CReSTeD list).

Adult Dyslexia & Skills Development Centre
(A,C,R,TC,TTC,Adults)
Dr D McLoughlin, London
Tel. 020 7388 8744
Fax. 020 7387 7968
dyslexia@adsdc.freeserve.co.uk

The American School in London (M)
Dr H I Jackson, London
Tel. 020 7449 1204
Fax. 020 7449 1357
Helen_Jackson@asl.org

Ann Arbor, Publishers Ltd. (B)
Mr P Laverack, Northumberland
Tel. 01668 214 581
Fax. 01668 214 484
enquiries@annarbor.co.uk
www.annarbor.co.uk

Appleford School (R,S)
Mr P Stanley, Wiltshire
Tel. 01980 621 020
Fax. 01980 621 366
secretary@appleford.demon.co.uk

Arts Dyslexia Trust (Hon)
Mrs S Parkinson, Kent
Tel. 01303 813 221
Fax. 01303 813 221
ArtsDysT@aol.com
www.sniffout.net/home/adt

Aston House Dyslexia Consultancy
(A,C,R)
Dr M Newton, Worcs
Tel. 01684 567 422

Avon House School & Dyslexia Centre (A,M,TC)
Ms F Cookson, Essex
Tel. 020 8504 1749

B/E Business & Education Consultancy (A,R,TC Adults)
Mrs J Byatt, Shropshire
Tel: 0169˙ 623 644
Fax: 0169 623 614
be.consult@btinternet.com

Bangor Dyslexia Unit (A,B,HE,R,TC TTC incl adults)
Mrs M Jones, Gwynedd
Tel. 01248 382 203
Fax. 01248 383 614
m.jones@bangor.ac.uk.
www.dyslexia.bangor.ac.uk/

Beaudesert Park School (M)
Mrs K Duffy, Gloucestershire
Tel. 01453 832 072
Fax: 01453 836 040
office@beaudesert.org.uk
www.beaudesert.org.uk

The Bebbington Dyslexia Centre
(A,TC)
Mr A Hargreaves, Cumbria
Tel. 01539 433 419

Bedgebury School
Mrs H Moriarty, Kent
Tel. 01580 211 221
Fax: 01580 212 252
info@bedgebury.ndirect.co.uk
www.bedgebury,ndirect.co.uk

Beechwood Sacred Heart (M)
Mrs V Letchworth, Kent
Tel. 01892 532 747

Better Books (B)
Mr P Wilkes, Worcs
Tel. 01384 253 276
Fax. 01384 253 285
sales@betterbooks.co.uk
www.dyslexiabooks.co.uk

Blossom House School (S)
Mrs J Burgess, London.
Tel. 020 8946 7348
Fax. 020 8944 5848
blossom.house@appleonline.net

Bloxham School (M)
Mr H J Alexander, Oxfordshire
Tel. 01295 720 222
Fax. 01295 721 714
hughalexander@talk21.com
www.bloxham.oxon.sch.uk

Bredon School (A,M,TC)
Mrs S E West, Gloucestershire
Tel. 01684 293 156
Fax. 01684 298 008
enquiries@bredonschool.co.uk
www.boarding-schools.com

**Bristol Dyslexia Centre & Belgrave
School** (A, C, S, TC incl adults)
Mrs P Jones, Bristol
Tel. 0117 973 9405
Fax. 0117 923 9703
pat@dyslexiacentre.co.uk
www.dyslexiacentre.co.uk

Broxbourne Dyslexia Unit
(A,C, TC,TTC incl adults)
Mrs G Westcombe, Herts
Tel. 01992 442 002
Fax. 01992 442 002

Bruern Abbey School (S)
Mr J Stirling Stover, Oxon
Tel. 01869 242 448
Fax. 01869 243 949
secretary@bruernabbey.org

Calder House School (S)
Mr C Agombar, Wilts
Tel. 01225 742 329
Fax. 01225 742 329

Cameron House (M)
Mrs Ouida, London
Tel. 020 7352 4040
Fax. 020 7352 2349
cameronhouse@lineone.net

Carmarthenshire College
(A, FE, HE, TC,TTC)
Mr R G Davies, Llanelli
Tel. 01554 748 000
Fax. 01554 756 088
Robert.Davies@ccta.ac.uk
www.ccta.ac.uk

Centre Academy (A,C,R,S,TC,TTC)
Mr F O'Regan, London
Tel. 020 7738 2344
Fax. 020 7738 9862
ukadmin@centreacademy.com
www.centeracademy.com

Child Consultants (A,C,R)
Mr P Kendall, London
Tel. 020 7637 3177
Fax. 020 7637 3181
jeni@childconsultants.com
www.childconsultants.com

City College Birmingham
(FE,HE,Adults)
Mrs L Parkinson, Birmingham
Tel. 0121 256 1072

City of Bath College (FE, Adults)
Mr D Symington, Bath
Tel. 01225 328 653
symingtond@citybathcoll.ac.uk

Class Consultants
(A,C,R,TC incl adults)
Mrs R Bolter, Monmouthshire
Tel. 01873 855 130
Fax: 01873 855 130
ruthbolter@class-consultants.co.uk
www.class-consultants.co.uk

Cobham Hall (M)
Mrs C A Ostler, Kent
Tel. 01474 823 371
Fax. 01474 825 902
ushered@cobhamhall.com
www.cobhamhall.com

Colston's Collegiate Lower School
(M) Mrs N J Whitaker, Bristol
Tel. 0117 965 5297

Connaught House Dyslexia Centre
(A,M,TC)
Mrs Fowke, Kent
Tel. 01305 785 703
Fax. 01305 780 976
admin@thornlow.co.uk
www.thornlow.co.uk

Delamere Forest School (S)
Mrs J Vegoda, Cheshire
Tel. 01928 788 263
Fax. 01928 788 263

Deptford Green School (M)
Mrs C Barry, London
Tel. 020 8691 3236
Fax. 020 8694 1789

The Dominie (S)
Ms L Robertson, London
Tel. 020 7720 8783
Fax. 020 7720 8783
LRDominie@aol.com

Dyslexia Advisory Bureau (A)
Dr R M Griffiths, Surrey
Tel. 01252 793 067
Fax. 01252 793 067

Dyslexia Association of Hong Kong
Mr J Gadbury, Hong Kong
Fax. 00 852 2872 5489
gadbury@iohk.com

Dyslexia Association of Ireland
(was ACLD) (A,C,TC,TTC incl adults)
Mrs A Hughes. Ireland
Tel. 01 679 0276
Fax. 01 679 0273
acld@iol.ie   www.acld-dyslexia.com

Dyslexia Institute (A,B,C,R,TC,TTC
incl adults)
Ms K Bennett, 23 Centres
Tel. 01784 463 851
Fax. 01784 460 747
info@dyslexia-inst.org.uk
www.dyslexia-inst.org.uk

**Dyslexia North West & Lancashire
Centre for SpLD(Dyslexia)**
(A,S,TC,TTC)
Mr C Lannen, Lancashire
Tel. 01253 720 570
Fax: 01253 720 570
colin.lannen@btinternet.com

Dyslexia Teaching Centre
(A,TC incl adults)
Mr A Stokes, London
Tel. 020 7937 2408
Fax. 020 7938 4816

East Court School (A,C,R,S)
Dr M E Thomson, Kent
Tel. 01843 592 077
Fax. 01843 592 418
dyslexia@eastcourtschool.co.uk
www.eastcourtschool.co.uk

Eaton House School (M)
Miss L Watts, London
Tel. 020 7730 9343
Fax: 020 7730 1798
EatonHse@aol.com

Edington & Shapwick School (A,S)
Mr D Walker, Somerset
Tel. 01278 722 012
Fax. 01278 723 312
edington@burtle.globalnet.co.uk
www.edingtonshapwick.co.uk

Ellesmere College (M)
Mr B Wignall, Shropshire
Tel. 01691 622 321
Fax. 01691 623 286

Ercall Wood Comprehensive School
Mr J Lewis, Shropshire
Tel. 01952 417 800
Fax. 01952 417 803

Fairley House School (S)
Ms A Fitzgerald, London
Tel. 020 7976 5456
Fax. 020 7976 5905
office@fairleyhouse.westminster.sch.uk

Frewen College (S)
Mr S Horsley, East Sussex,
Tel. 01797 252 494
Fax. 01797 252 567
post@frewcoll.demon.co.uk
www.frewcoll.demon.co.uk

David Fulton (Publishers) Ltd (B)
Mr D Fulton, London.
Tel. 020 7405 5606
Fax. 020 7831 4840
david.fulton@fultonbooks.co.uk
www.fultonbooks.co.uk

Grenville College (M)
Dr M C V Cane, North Devon
Tel. 01237 472 212   Fax. 01237 477 020
info@grenville.devon.sch.uk
www.grenville.devon.sch.uk

Dr G Hales (A,C incl adults)
Milton Keynes
Tel. 01908 312 880
Fax. 01908 317 691
drghales@aol.com

Hawkhurst Court Dyslexia Centre
(M) Mr D Ollosson, Brighton
Tel. 01273 704 218
Fax: 01273 704 331
dyslexia@brightoncollege.org.uk
www.brightoncollege.demon.co.uk

Helen Arkell Dyslexia Centre
(A,B,TC,TTC incl Adults)
Mrs R Wood, Surrey
Tel. 01252 792 400
Fax. 01252 795 669
general_enquiries@arkellcentre.org.uk
www.arkellcentre.org.uk

Hillcroft Preparatory School
(A,C,M,TC)
Mrs G Rapsey, Suffolk
Tel. 01449 673 003

**Hornsby International Dyslexia
Centre** (A,B,TTC, incl adults)
Mr J Dixon, London
Tel. 020 7223 1144
Fax. 020 7924 1112
dyslexia@hornsby.co.uk
www.hornsby.co.uk

HQ Directorate of Educational & Training Services (Army) (FE)
Major M Claridge, Wilts
Tel. 01980618714
Fax. 01980 618 705
dets_a@gtnet.gov.uk

iANSYST Ltd (A,B,C,R incl adult)
Mr I Litterick, Cambridge
Tel. 01223 420 101
Fax. 01223 426 644
sales@dyslexic.com
www.dyslexic.com

Jean Norton Trust Fund (A,R,TC)
Mrs J Norton MBE, Essex
Tel. 01268 710 200

Kingham Hill School (M)
Mrs S Shorter, Oxford
Tel. 01608 658 999
Fax. 01608 658 658
admissions@kingham-hill.oxon.sch.uk
www.kingham-hill.oxon.sch.uk

Kings' College School (M)
Mrs L Chapman, Cambridge
Tel. 01223 365 814
Fax: 0122 461 388
hm@kingscam.demon.co.uk

King's School
Mrs V Trenchard, Somerset
Tel: 01749 814 200
Fax. 01749 813 326
kingshm@kingsbruton.somerset.sch.uk
www.kingsbruton.com

Knowl Hill School (S)
Mrs A Bareford, Surrey
Tel. 01483 797 032
Fax. 01483 797 641
ajb@knowlhill.surrey.sch.uk
www.knowlhill.org.uk

Laleham School (S)
Mrs F Lewis, Margate
Tel. 01843 221 946
Fax. 01843 231 368
felicitylewis@laleham.kent.sch.uk

LDA Living & Learning (B)
Ms G Griffin, Cambridge
Tel. 01223 357 744
Fax. 01223 460 557
ldaorders@compuserve.com
www.instructionalfair.co.uk

Learning Curve Associates
(Educational Consultants)
(C,FE,HE,TTC,Adults)
Mrs V Mackenzie, Bucks
Tel. 01753 643 149
Fax. 01753 643 149
val@learning-curve.demon.co.uk
www.learning-curve.org

Learning Solutions
(A,C,R,TC,TTC incl adults)
Mr A Heath, Bradford
Tel. 01274 777 250
Fax. 01274 778 754
alan@learning-solutions.co.uk
www.learning-solutions.co.uk

Learning Support Service (Kingston Upon Thames) (A,TC,TTC)
Mrs D Da Silva
Tel. 020 8546 3389
Fax. 020 8974 5416
learning.support@rbk.kingston.gov.uk

Learning Support Service (Newham)
Ms P Corr, London
Tel. 020 8555 5552
Fax. 020 8557 6003

**Literacy Assessment & Research
Centre** (A,C,FE,HE,R,TC,TTC Adults)
Dr E Doctor, London
Tel. 020 7612 6416
Fax. 020 7612 6427
eadoctor@aol.com

Manchester Metropolitan University
(A,C,HE,R,TC,TTC)
Mrs S Phillips, Manchester
Tel: 0161 247 2051
Fax: 0161 247 6368
s.phillips@mmu.ac.uk

**Maple Hayes Dyslexia School &
Resource Centre** (A,R,S)
Dr E N Brown, Staffordshire
Tel. 01543 264 387
Fax:01543 262 022
brown-dr@dyslexia-
maplehayes.staffs.sch.uk
www.dyslexia.gb.com

Mark College (S)
Mrs J Kay, Somerset
Tel. 01278 641 632
Fax. 01278 641 426
post@markcollege.org.uk

Mayville High School (M)
Ms L Owens, Hampshire
Tel. 023 9273 4847
Fax. 023 9229 3649
mayvillehighschool@talk21.com

Medway Dyslexia Centre
(A,TC,TTC incl adults)
Mr J H Sears, Kent
Tel. 01634 848 232
Fax. 01634 818 787
strathdee@cableinet.co.uk
www.medwaydyslexiacentre.co.uk

Millfield Preparatory School (M)
Mr D Hopkin, Somerset
Tel. 01458 832 446
Fax. 01458 833 679
office@millfieldprep.somerset.sch.uk
www.millfield.somerset.sch.uk/prep

Millfield School (M)
Mrs M McGlone, Somerset
Tel. 01458 442 291
Fax. 01458 447 276
dmm@millfield.somerset.sch.uk
www.millfield.somerset.sch.uk

The Moat School (S)
Mr R Carlysle, London
Tel. 020 7610 9018
Fax. 020 7610 9098
moatsch@pavilion.co.uk
www.pavilion.co.uk/moatsch

Moon Hall School (S)
Mrs J Lovett, Surrey
Tel. 01306 731 464
Fax. 01306 731 504
enquiries@moonhall.surrey.sch.uk
www.moonhall.surrey.sch.uk

More House School
Mr B Huggett, Surrey
Tel. 01252 792 303
Fax. 01252 797 601
morehouseschool@hotmail.com

Multi Sensory Learning Ltd (B)
Ms P Attwood
Tel. 01536 399 003
Fax. 01536 399 012
FirstBest9@aol.com

New Eccles Hall School
Mr R Allard, Norfolk
Tel. 01953 887 217
Fax: 10953 887 397
nehs@quidenham.freeserve.co.uk
www.quidenham.freeserve.co.uk

New Hope Special School
(A,C,R,S,TTC)
Dr E Rossides, Cyprus
Tel: 00 357 2 494 820
Fax:. 00 357 2 427 928
newhope@rossides.com
www.rossides.com

New Learning Centre (A,C,S)
Mrs N Janis-Norton, London
Tel. 020 7794 0321
Fax. 020 7431 8600
tnlc@dial.pipex.com

Next Generation
(A,B,C,R,TC,TTC incl adults)
Ms J Poustie, Somerset
Tel. 01823 289 559
Fax. 01823 289 559
jan.poustie@virgin.net
www.janpoustie.co.uk

Northbrook FE and HE College
(FE,HE,TTC,Adults)
Mr M Whinney, West Sussex
Tel. 01903 606 060
Fax. 01903 606 007
enquiries@nbcol.ac.uk
www.nbcol.ac.uk

Northease Manor School (C,S,TTC)
Mr R J Dennien, Sussex
Tel. 01273 472 915
Fax. 01273 472 202
northease@msn.com
www.northeasemanor.e-sussex.sch.uk

Nunnykirk Hall School (S)
Mr S Dalby-Ball, Northumberland
Tel. 01670 772 685
Fax. 01670 772 434
secretary@nkirk.freeserve.co.uk

The Old Rectory School (S)
Mr T R Smith, Suffolk
Tel. 01449 736 404
Fax. 01449 737 881
oldrectoryschool@talk21.com

The Oldham College (A,FE Adults)
Mrs M Dixon, Oldham
Tel: 0161 624 5214
Fax: 0161 785 4234
mary.dixon@oldham.ac.uk

PATOSS The Professional Ass'n of Teachers of Students with SpLD
Worcs
Fax. 01386 712 640
patoss@evesham.ac.uk
www.patoss-dyslexia.org

Ramillies Hall School (M)
Mrs A L Poole, Cheshire
Tel. 0161 485 3804
Fax. 0161 485 6021
Ramillies@btinternet.com

Ryde School (M)
Mrs A Mellor, Isle of Wight
Tel. 01983 562 229
Fax: 01983 564 714
headmaster@rydeschool.org.uk
www.rydeschool.org.uk

Scottish Dyslexia Trust
Mr A Maclay, Edinburgh
Tel. 01835 823 003
Fax. 01835 823 003
Agmaclay@aol.com
www.dyslexia-scotland.org.uk

SEMERC Information Service/Granada Learning (B,C)
Mr J R Hughes, Manchester
Tel. 0161 827 2719
Fax. 0161 827 2966
sis@granadamedia.com
www.semerc.com

SEN Marketing (Special Needs Bookshop) (B)
Mr C Redman, Wakefield
Tel. 01924 871 697
Fax. 01924 871 697
sen.marketing@ukonline.co.uk
www.sen.uk.com

SENS City & County of Swansea (C,R,TTC)
Mr C Warwick, Swansea
Tel. 01792 405 689
Fax. 01792 404 705
team@sensswansea.freeserve.co.uk

Sibford School (M)
Mrs S Freestone, Oxfordshire
Tel. 01295 781 200
Fax. 01295 781 204
sibford.school@dial.pipex.com
www.sibford.oxon.sch.uk

South Trafford College (FE)
Mrs J Harland, Cheshire
Tel. 0161 952 4755
Fax. 0161 952 4672
jharland@stcoll.ac.uk
www.stcoll.ac.uk

Special Needs Computing (B)
Ms J Simmons, Merseyside
Tel. 0151 426 9988
Fax. 051 426 9994
info@box42.com

St Bees School
Mrs J Wharrier, Cumbria
Tel. 01946 822 263
Fax. 01946 823 657
mailbox@st-bees-school.co.uk
www.st-bees-school.co.uk

St David's College (S)
Mr W Seymour, North Wales
Tel. 01492 875 974
Fax 01492 870 383
www.stdavidscollege.co.uk

Stanbridge Earls School (A,M,R)
Mr H Moxon, Hampshire
Tel. 01794 516 777
Fax. 01794 511 201
stanearls@aol.com

Stockport College (A,FE,HE)
Mr S Russell, Stockport
Tel. 0161 958 3425
Fax. 0161 480 3384
dyslexia@stockport.ac.uk
www.stockport.ac.uk

Swindon Dyslexia Centre (A,B,C,TC)
Mrs M Chivers, Wiltshire
Tel. 01793 433 967
Fax: 01793 433 967
maria-chivers@swindon-dyslexia-centre.fsbusiness.co.uk
www.DyslexiaA2Z.com

Tintavision (B,R)
Mr P Irons, Peterborough
Tel. 01778 349 233
Fax: 01778 349 244
enquiries@tintavision.com
www.tintavision.com

Touch-Type, Read and Spell (TC)
Mr P Alexandre, Kent
Tel: 020 8464 1330
Fax:020 8313 9454
p.alexandre@ttrs.co.uk
www.ttrs.co.uk

Wessex Dyslexia Tutors Group (TC)
Mrs E Hamilton, Dorset
Tel. 01202 698 617

White Space Ltd. (B)
Ms T Wahnon, London
Tel. 020 8748 5927
Fax. 020 8748 5927
sales@wordshark.co.uk
www.wordshark.co.uk

Wolverhampton Grammar School
Dr B Trafford, Dorset
Tel. 01902 421 326
Fax. 01902 421 819
wgs@wgs.org.uk

CReSTeD Schools

The Council for the Registration of Schools Teaching Dyslexic Pupils

(In "Type" M=Mixed, B= Boys only, G=Girls only)

Category SP Schools (Formerly Category A - See page 57 for guidance)

	Telephone	Pupils	Type	Ages
Appleford School				
Shrewton, Salisbury, Wiltshire, SP3 4HL	01980 621020	90	M	7-13
Brown's School				
Cannock House, Hawstead Lane, Chelsfield, BR6 7PH	01689 876816	33	M	6-12
Calder House School				
Colerne, Bath, Wiltshire, SN14 8BN	01225 742329	32	M	5-13
Centre Academy				
92 St John,s Hill, Battersea, London SW11 1SH	0207 738 2344	55	M	8-18
Dominie (The)				
142 Battersea Park Road, Battersea, London, SW11 4NB				
	020 7720 8783	32	M	6-13
East Court School				
Victoria Parade, Ramsgate, Kent, CT11 8ED	01843 592077	67	M	8-13
Edington & Shapwick School				
Shapwick Manor, Shapwick, Bridgwater, Somerset, TA9 9NJ				
	01458 210384	169	M	8-17
Fairley House School				
30 Causton Street, London, SW1P 4AU	020 7976 5456	95	M	6-12
Frewen College				
Brickwall, Northiam, Rye, Sussex, TN31 6NL	01797 252494	69	B	11-17
Knowl Hill School				
School Lane, Pirbright, Surrey, GU24 0JN	01483 797032	40	M	7-16
Laleham School				
Northdown Park Road, Cliftonville, Margate, Kent, CT9 2TP				
	01843 221946	104	M	9-16
Mark College				
Mark, Highbridge, Somerset, TA9 4NP	01278 641632	80	B	11-16
Moon Hall School				
Feldemore, Holmbury St Mary, Dorking, Surrey RH5 6LQ				
	01306 731464	80	M	7-13
More House School				
Moons Hill, Frensham, Farnham, Surrey, GU10 3AP	01252 792303	150	B	9-16

	Telephone	Pupils	Type	Ages
New Hope Private Special School 16 Kimonos Street, Acropolis, PO Box 28767, Nicosia 2082, Cyprus	+357 2 494820	57	M	6-17
Northease Manor School Rodmell, Lewes, Sussex, BN7 3EY	01273 472915	85	M	10-17
Nunnykirk Centre for Dyslexia Netherwitton, Morpeth, Northumberland NE61 4PB	01670 772685	40	M	9-16
Old Rectory School (The) Brettenham, Ipswich, Suffolk IP7 7QR	01449 736404	48	M	7-13
Sunnydown School Portley House, 152 Whyteleafe Road, Caterham, Surrey CR3 5ED	01883 342281	74	B	11-16
Unicorn School (The) Stroud Court, Oxford Road, Eynsham, Oxfordshire OX8 1BY	01865 881820	36	M	6-12

Category DU Schools (Formerly Category B - See page 57 for guidance)

	Telephone	Pupils	Type	Ages
Abbotsholme School Rocester, Uttoxeter, Staffordshire ST14 5BS	01889 590217	235	M	9-18
Avon House School 490 High Road, Woodford Green, Essex IG8 0PN	0181 504 1749	250	M	2.5-11
Bethany School Curtisden Green, Goudhurst, Cranbrook, Kent TN17 1LB	01580 211273	280	M	11-18
Bloxham School Bloxham, Banbury, Oxfordshire OX15 4PE	01295 720222	385	M	11-18
Clayesmore Preparatory School Iwerne Minster, Blandford Forum, Dorset DT11 8PH	01747 811707	260	M	5-13
Clayesmore School Iwerne Minster, Blandford Forum, Dorset DT11 8LL	01747 812122	305	M	13-18
Clifton College Preparatory School The Avenue, Clifton, Bristol BS8 3HE	0117 973 7264	400	M	8-13
Cobham Hall School Cobham, Kent DA12 3BL	01474 823371	190	G	11-18
Ellesmere College Ellesmere, Shropshire SY12 9AB	01691 622321	410	M	9-18

	Telephone	Pupils	Type	Ages
Ercall Wood Technology College Golf Links Lane, Wellington, Telford, Shropshire TF1 2DU	01952 417800	825	M	11-16
Fulneck School Fulneck, Pudsey, Leeds, West Yorkshire LS28 8DS	0113 257 0235	424	M	3-18
Grenville College Bideford, Devon EX39 3JR	01237 472212	380	M	8-18
Hillcroft Preparatory School Walnutree Manor, Haughley Green, Stowmarket, Suffolk IP14 3RQ	01449 673003	86	M	2-13
Holmwood House School Lexden, Colchester, Essex CO3 5ST	01206 574305	338	M	4-13
Hurst Lodge Bagshot Road, Ascot, Berkshire SL5 9JU	01344 622154	200	M	2.5-18
Kingham Hill School Kingham, Chipping Norton, Oxfordshire OX7 6TH	01608 658999	210	M	11-18
King's School Rochester Satis House, Boley Hill, Rochester, Kent ME1 1TE	01634 843913	340	M	13-18
King's School Rochester Preparatory School King Edward Road, Rochester, Kent ME1 1UB	01634 843657	230	M	8-13
Merchiston Castle School Colinton, Edinburgh EH13 0PU Scotland	0131 312 2200	390	B	8-18
New Hall School Chelmsford, Essex CM3 3HT	01245 467588	650	M	4-18
Newlands Preparatory School Eastbourne Road, Seaford, Sussex BN25 4NP	01323 892334	200	M	7-13
Pocklington School West Green, Pocklington, Yorkshire YO42 2NJ	01759 303125	750	M	7-18
Roundhay School Gledhow Lane, Leeds LS8 1ND	0113 293 7711	1192	M	11-18
St David's College Llandudno, Conwy, LL30 1RD, Wales	01492 875974	210	M	11-18
St James's School West Malvern, Worcestershire WR14 4DF	01684 560851	120	G	10-18
Sibford School Sibford Ferris, Banbury, Oxfordshire OX15 5QL	01295 781200	320	M	5-18
Sidcot School Winscombe, Somerset BS25 1PD	01934 843102	480	M	3-18

Stanbridge Earls School
Romsey, Hampshire, SO51 0ZS   01794 516777   184   M   11-18

Stowford College
95 Brighton Road, Sutton, Surrey SM2 5SJ   020 8661 9444   70   M   7-16+

Thornlow Preparatory School
Connaught Road, Weymouth, Dorset DT4 0SA   01305 785703   70   M   3-13

Category SC Schools (Formerly Category C - See page 57 for guidance)

	Telephone	Pupils	Type	Ages
Bodiam Manor School Bodiam, Robertsbridge, East Sussex TN32 5UJ	01580 830225	170	M	2-13
Box Hill School Mickleham, Dorking, Surrey RH5 6EA	01372 373382	268	M	11-18
Bronte House School Apperley Bridge, Bradford, Yorkshire BD10 0PQ	0113 250 2811	303	M	3-11
Danes Hill School Leatherhead Road, Oxshott, Surrey KT22 0JG	01372 842509	800	M	3-13
Hugh Christie Technology College Norwich Avenue, Tonbridge, Kent TN10 4QL 01732 353544/358288		1100	M	11-18
King's School Ely Ely, Cambridgeshire CB7 4DB	01353 660700	400	M	13-18
King's School Junior School Ely, Cambridgeshire CB7 4DB	01353 660730	320	M	8-13
Llandovery College Llandovery, Carmarthenshire, SA20 0EE, Wales	01550 723000	220	M	11-18
Mayville High School 35 St Simon's Road, Southsea, Hampshire PO5 2PE	01705 734847	250	M	4-16
Mount St Mary's College Spinkhill, Derbyshire S21 3YL	01246 433388	285	M	11-18
Newlands Manor Senior School Eastbourne Road, Seaford, Sussex BN25 4NP	01323 890309	160	M	13-18
Newlands Pre-Preparatory & Nursery School Eastbourne Road, Seaford, Sussex BN25 1JW	01323 896461	149	M	2.5-8
Ramillies Hall School Cheadle Hulme, Cheadle, Cheshire SK8 7AJ	0161 485 3804	89	M	4-13
Slindon College Slindon House, Slindon, Arundel, Sussex BN18 0RH	01243 814320	110	B	10-16
St Elphin's School Darley Dale, Matlock, Derbyshire DE4 2HA	01629 733263	135	G	5-16

Category WS Schools (Formerly Category D - See page 57 for guidance)

	Telephone	Pupils	Type	Ages
Hordle Walhampton School Lymington, Hampshire SO41 5ZG	01590 672013	177	M	7-13
Monkton Combe School Monkton Combe, Bath, Avon BA2 7HG	01225 721102	346	M	11-18
Mowden Hall School Newton, Stocksfield, Northumberland NE43 7TP	01661 842147	170	M	4-13
Newlands School 34 The Grove, Gosforth, Newcastle upon Tyne NE3 1NH 0191 285 2208	0191 285 2208	210	B	3-13
Prior Park Preparatory School Calcutt Street, Cricklade, Wiltshire SN6 6BB	01793 750275	187	M	7-13
St Bede's School Bishton Hall, Wolseley Bridge, Staffordshire ST17 0XN 01889 881277	01889 881277	130	M	3-13
St Bees School St Bees, Cumbria CA27 0DS	01946 822263	300	M	11-18
Windlesham House School Washington, Pulborough, West Sussex RH20 4AY	01903 873207	290	M	4-13
Woodhouse Grove School Apperley Bridge, West Yorkshire BD10 0NR	0113 250 2477	555	M	11-16
Woodleigh School Langton Langton Hall, Langton, Malton, North Yorkshire YO17 9QN 01653 658215	01653 658215	55	M	7-13

SpLD courses for teachers

Centres whose courses include BDA accredited Specific Learning Difficulties/ Dyslexia training for teachers. Contact the centres for details of course contents, coursework required, the qualifications obtained and ask which of their courses are BDA accredited.

Bangor, University of Wales.
Gwen Hughes   Tel: 01248 382 932   Fax: 01248 383 092
E-mail: eds056@bangor.ac.uk   Web: www.bangor.ac.uk

Birmingham University.
Dr Lyn Layton   Tel: 0121 414 4871   Fax: 0121 414 4865
E-mail: l.layton@bham.ac.uk   Web: www.edu.bham.ac.uk

Bristol University West of England.
John Dwyfor-Davies Tel: 0117 344 4127   Fax: 0117 976 2146
E-mail: Rebecca.Shepeard@uwe.ac.uk Web: www.uwe.ac.uk

Cheltenham & Gloucester SpLD.
Dr Terri Passenger   Tel: 01242 532 862   Fax: 01242 532 895
E-mail: angelah@chelt.ac.uk

Conwy County Borough Council.
Jacqueline Döll   Tel: 01492 575 019

Cumbria County Council
Janet Pinney   Tel: 01229 774 967   Fax: 01229 774 967

Dyslexia Institute.
National Training Office   Tel: 01784 463 851   Fax: 01784 460 747
E-mail: mwardell@dyslexia-inst.org.uk Web: www.dyslexia-inst.org.uk

Durham County Council.
Mary Coffield   Tel: 01740 656 998   Fax: 01740 657 792
E-mail: mary.coffield@durham.gov.uk

East Sussex County Council
Joan Amos   Tel: 01825 764 177   Fax: 01825 768 661
E-mail: lss.uckfield@easynet.co.uk

Helen Arkell Dyslexia Centre. (Includes FE/HE Courses)
Courses Secretary   Tel: 01252 792 400   Fax: 01252 795 669
E-mail: general_enquiries@arkellcentre.org.uk Web: www.arkellcentre.org.uk

Hornsby International Dyslexia Centre.
Attendance courses   Tel: 020 7223 1144   Fax: 020 7924 1112
E-mail: courses@hornsby.co.uk   Web: www.hornsby.co.uk

Leicester University
Morag Hunter Carsch   Tel: 0116 252 3703   Fax: 0116 252 3653
E-mail: cmh16@le.ac.uk

Liverpool John Moores University.
Pat Mullins/Andrea Wall   Tel: 0151 231 5261   Fax: 0151 231 5338
E-mail: a.wall@livjm.ac.uk

Manchester Metropolitan University. (Includes FE/HE Courses)
Sylvia Phillips   Tel: 0161 247 2051   Fax: 0161 247 6368
E-mail: s.phillips@mmu.ac.uk   Web: www.did.stu.mmu.ac.uk

Moray House, University of Edinburgh.
Pamela Deponio   Tel: 0131 651 6232   Fax: 0131 651 6511
E-mail: pamela.deponio@ed.ac.uk

Newport University of Wales.
Val Miller   Tel: 01633 432 217   Fax: 01633 432 074

OCR Diploma/Certificate courses (Oxford, Cambridge and RSA).
37 Centres for SpLD Dip/Cert 70 for CLANSA for Learning Support
Assistants.
OCR Customer Information Bureau Tel. 024 7647 0033
E-mail: cib@ocr.org.uk   Web: www.ocr.org.uk

Rotherham Metropolitan Borough Council.
Deborah Connell,   Tel: 01709 556 940

Sittingbourne Community College
(Learning Support Assistant Courses Only)
Mrs A Saunders   Tel: 01795 472 449   Fax: 01795 470 332
E-mail: office@sitcomcol.kent.sch.co.uk

Southampton University.
Mr G A Price   Tel: 023 8059 2611   Fax: 023 8059 3556
E-mail: gap@soton.ac.uk

Swansea LEA. (Includes courses for Learning Support Assistants).
Deborah Avington   Tel: 01792 405 689   Fax: 01792 404 705
E-mail: sens.adviser.tm@swansea.gov.uk

Swansea, University of Wales.
Wendy Cunnah   Tel: 01792 205 678   Fax: 01792 298 499

Computer co-ordinators

*The BDA encourages Local Dyslexia Associations to appoint computer
co-ordinators, who can answer ICT enquiries and perhaps arrange talks and
workshops. If your area is not covered, please call the helpline of your nearest
Local Dyslexia Association (see pages 86-97).*

Local Dyslexia Association	Telephone	E-mail
Barnet DA	020 8441 7626	
Bedford DA	01234 211 071	
South Bedfordshire DA	01582 664 661	denise@dunstable.demon.co.uk
West Berkshire DA	0118 933 2858	
Birmingham DA	0121 633 9553	
Birmingham Adult DG	01827 51 506	PA.Smith@which.net
Bolton & District DA	01204 693 478	S.J.Singleton@btinternet.com
DA Bristol	0117 971 5927	julian@milby.freeserve.co.uk
Calderdale DA	01422 884 206	michaelairey@northvale.sagehost.co.uk
Cambridge DA	01223 860 142	
Cheshire DA	01270 651 301	
Cornwall DA	01872 571 038	sarahw@cockshill.fsnet.co.uk
Croydon DA	020 8660 1925	
North Cumbria DA	01228 670 205	
South Cumbria DA	01229 587 881	
West Cumbria DA	01946 725 202	
Darlington &DDSG	01325 263 750	
Devon DA	01803 852 004	
Dorset DA	01747 854 724	dhillage@argonet.co.uk
Dudley DA	01384 422 794	pstewart@halesowen.ac.uk
Ealing DA	020 8567 3400	rod.hawkins@dial.pipex.com
Enfield & District DA	020 8363 3178	ken@dibley-harper.freeserve.co.uk
Gloucestershire DA	01242 703 609	
Harrow SPELD	020 8954 6080	Nckaufman@aol.com
Hertfordshire DA	01582 620 957	chris.chall.ntlworld.com
Hillingdon DA	01895 672 617	hdahelpline@yahoo.co.uk
North Kent DA	020 8464 1330	p.alexandre@ttrs.co.uk
South Kent DA	01233 661 116	dyslexia.teacher.carol@mcphillimy.freeserve.co.uk
Kent West DA	01892 542 927	irene.heskett@virgin.net
Kingston DA	020 8390 6955	
Leeds & Bradford DA	01274 771 153	jane@labda.org.uk

Leicestershire DA	0116 270 2003	
Liverpool DA	0151 722 1029	Maureen-Wilcock@maureen-wilcock.freeserve.co.uk
London DA	020 7222 2784	AlanCot@btinternet.com
Medway DA	0961 334 561	barry@wjames.freeserve.co.uk
Merton & SW London DA	020 8785 1516	ann.hilton@virgin.net
Northamptonshire DA	01604 493 103	
Nottinghamshire DA	0115 955 5155	Deborah.Wheeldon@theNDA.fsnet.co.uk
Oxfordshire DA	01865 200 665	Bernard.Sufrin@comlab.ox.ac.uk
Peterborough & District DA	01778 341 719	KevinTaylor@northborough.freeserve.co.uk
Rugby & District DA	024 7654 2385	101650.3570@compuserve.com
Rutland DA	01572 787 503	
Salford DA	0161 790 8701	Leather.Family@btinternet.com
Somerset DA	01458 210 524	anthbeale@aol.com
DA for N Somerset	01934 625 298	cpcjn@breathemail.net
Southport & District DA	01695 577 631	
St Helens DA	01744 24 608	dwylan@cwcom.net
Stockport DA	0161 440 0818	
Suffolk DA	01473 833 071	julian_k@anglianet.co.uk
East Sussex DA	01323 896 542	nicky@woodward3040.freeserve.co.uk
West Sussex DA	01903 211 965	wsda@cwcom.net
Sutton DA	020 8715 7844	Dazmoh1@blueyonder.co.uk
Trafford DA	0161 775 7870	
Central Tyneside DA	0191 455 5954	Judith@wolfe83.freeserve.co.uk
Wakefield & District DA	01977 511 581	dyslexia@cclc.co.uk
DA for Walsall Now [DAWN]	01922 867 764	dawndyslexia@yahoo.com
North Warwickshire DA	024 7638 2263	
Waveney Valley DA	01603 715 649	
Wigan & District DA	01257 423 246	
Wiltshire DA	01373 830 411	
DA of Windsor & Maidenhead, Slough, Bracknell	01628 631 794	suepv@lineone.net
DA [Wirral]	0151 645 9946	
Gwent DA	01291 627 034	chris.sharp@dial.pipex.com
West Wales DA	01792 201 776	M.C.Sykes@swan.ac.uk
Jersey DA	01534 853 086	

Dyslexia Worldwide

BDA covers England, Wales and Northern Ireland. However, it holds a list which contains at least one contact for each of the following countries:

Australia	Hong Kong	Norway
Austria	India	Pakistan
Belgium	Indonesia	Puerto Rico
Brazil	Israel	Russia
Canada	Japan	Singapore
Cyprus	Kenya	South Africa
Czech Republic	Kuwait	Spain
Denmark	Lebanon	Sweden
Dubai (Abu Dhabi)	Luxembourg	Switzerland
Eire	Malta	United Arab Emirates
France	Netherlands	USA
Germany	New Zealand	Zimbabwe
Greece	Nigeria	

For other countries, you may like to ask the Hornsby International Dyslexia Centre for a list of teachers who have undertaken the distance learning courses for teachers (correspondence courses). Tel: 020 7223 1144 Fax: 020 7924 1112. E-mail: dyslexia@hornsby.co.uk   Web: www.hornsby.co.uk

Another contact is Ian Smythe, Handbook editor and co-editor of the International Book of Dyslexia. As well as the above, he also has links with the following countries: Argentina, Bulgaria, Chile, China, Croatia, Finland, Hungary, Iceland, Italy, Jordan, Malaysia, Namibia, Peru, Philippines, Poland, Slovakia, Slovenia, and Thailand with some details of which are on the web site below. Tel: 0208 770 0888   Fax: 0208 770 0936 E-mail: ian.smythe@ukonline.co.uk Web: http://web.ukonline.co.uk/wdnf

The European Dyslexia Association and International Dyslexia Association may also be able to provide further contacts. See their articles in Section 1.

Part 3 - Managing dyslexia

This section contains chapters on ways to cope with dyslexia, whether you are a parent, a teacher or a dyslexic person in the adult world; on obtaining special provision for dyslexic children; and suggestions for further reading.

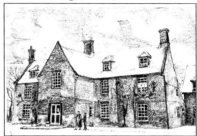

Meeting the Social and Emotional Needs of Gifted and Talented Dyslexic Children

Lindsay Peer, Education Director, British Dyslexia Association

There is a great deal that needs to be done on the recognition of and support for dyslexic people who are gifted. In this article I use the term giftedness to describe children who have outstanding ability in specific areas of the curriculum, far and beyond those of their peers. The Code of Practice (DfEE) does not recognise giftedness as a special need; it does recognise dyslexia. Education Authorities and schools often see dyslexic weaknesses as measured by the class average. For the dyslexic learner this is far from acceptable. For them, the gap between what they should be able to achieve and what they do achieve is the critical issue. In The Report of the Working Party on Dyslexia in Higher Education (1998), it is stated that:

'Intellectual potential, represented by the abilities of individuals, is a social, cultural and economic asset that no nation can afford to neglect. Equal opportunities and anti-discrimination legislation encourage the entry of talented but disabled students into higher education. When the existence of a legally – recognised disability such as dyslexia obscures the recognition of able individuals by institutions of higher education, the individual, educational institutions and the nation lose.'

The Common Link

There are many examples of gifted adults who are also dyslexic, proving that the two conditions co-exist. Some people find that notion strange, but it is indisputable. They are both

'invisible disabilities' which have much in common. Both:

- make the child feel 'different'

- cause 'important others' to relate to them in ways not suited to their needs

- cause the growing child to develop differently from their friends

- may cause social and emotional difficulties.

Gifted dyslexic learners can think, talk and reason perfectly well. They may however have significant difficulty reading and/or expressing their highly developed ideas on paper. They will often be aware that there are other learners about them who cannot think and reason to anywhere near the same level. They see the unfairness when they receive low marks due to the low level of their literacy skills and their less able peers receive higher marks as they have 'written better'.

To achieve full academic, social and emotional potential, a high level of motivation and self-esteem has to be maintained throughout the long number of years spent at school. Under this pressure, there are many circumstances that might cause gifted dyslexic people to drop out along the way. What a loss to us all!

The gifted child can reason, perform, understand and talk about their area of excellence at adult level, but still be a child emotionally and socially. Adults often do not know how to handle such contrasts in gifted young people - particularly if they are dyslexic too. Both giftedness and dyslexia can affect the way children think about themselves; how they 'fit' into their peer group and what kind of person they may ultimately become.

Another area of similarity is that of adult decision making. For example if a child shows outstanding musical ability, ideally competent tuition and extensive practice should take place

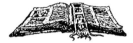
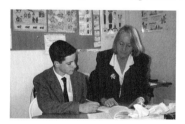

from a very young age. An adult must decide whether this will or will not happen. A similar situation will occur if a child shows dyslexic-type difficulties. Structured, sequential, multi-sensory teaching together with skills development will need to be put into place as early as possible. If this does not happen, the child may well fall behind at school. Dependence therefore on adult decision making is critical for these children. If parents and teachers are not empowered and knowledgeable, even the gifts of creativity and thinking can be lost leaving learners frustrated, unsupported and highly vulnerable.

The very existence of both conditions has been a matter of heated debate until quite recently. The word 'belief' was even used in relation to both of them. What is dyslexia? Can a condition exist if you cannot see it? What is giftedness? How do we identify both conditions? Do we treat such children in the same way as others? Are they special needs children? Could the two conditions really exist side by side? There are many overlaps and a great need to ensure that: (a) educators are trained, (b) the public is aware and (c) that appropriate policy is in place at local and national level.

Dyslexia and giftedness are now grounded on a much firmer research and practice basis. In the 1970s, Geschwind, an eminent researcher and the founder of the Harvard Medical Centre for the study of the brains of dyslexics wrote about their relatedness. He suggested that the specific construction of the dyslexic brain '...may explain the superior right hemisphere capacities exhibited by dyslexic children." He also identified learners with hyperlexia, who despite apparent ability in reading aloud, comprehended at a low level. What is clear and exciting is that Geschwind's initial notion of highly able right hemispheric learners has been borne out. There is much evidence that many dyslexic learners may have high abilities in the visual and creative fields. (West, 1991.) We need only look at the colleges of art and design; at the university departments

producing superb dyslexic dramatists, architects and engineers. They are all highly able, creative learners developing their abilities and adopting strategies to cope with their difficulties.

Identification and Remediation:

When using IQ tests to identify these children, results often show a disparity of ability between verbal and performance scores. They will often display one area or the other as being particularly high. The results should lead to an understanding of the child's learning styles and to an appropriate type of provision. It is vitally important for gifted dyslexic children that there is a balanced approach in both promoting strengths and in recognising and supporting difficulties. We need to address many areas of support which go far beyond the basic literacy and numeracy processes. Provision needs to cover the traditional areas of dyslexia weaknesses including:

- speed of processing
- organisation
- memory skills
- sequencing
- laterality

These lead to significant difficulties coping with the curriculum despite high ability.

For those in the gifted dyslexia group, there is an additional pressure, that of a need for perfectionism. There is direct conflict here where many dyslexic youngsters find themselves unable to reach the level that they so badly need. If perfectionism refers to having high standards, a desire to achieve, conscientiousness, or high levels of responsibility, it is likely to become a virtue, not a problem. However, it is a problem when it frustrates and inhibits achievement. Teachers must therefore be aware of the need to direct and support so that frustration and obsession do not set in.

It is critical that such children are identified as early on as is possible. There are tests now available that can identify children at risk of dyslexia as early as three years old. We no longer have to wait until children fall behind and their self-esteem plummets. What is vital is that alongside the early identification process is a programme that develops the pathways leading to effective learning. Multi-sensory teaching programmes have proven themselves internationally over many years and can be used to teach reading, spelling, grammar, punctuation as well as foreign languages and numeracy. For the older learner, programmes developing metacognitive processes and study skills programmes must be put into place, as the academic demands become weightier.

It is vital that teachers and specialists monitor the progress that is made by these children on a regular basis so as to ensure that realistic targets are being met. The brighter the child the higher the expectation should be. It is unacceptable to expect that the target for a gifted child to be at the level of the class average.

Policy in the UK currently requires that Special Educational Needs are recognised and that Individual/Group Education Plans are developed to answer need. Differentiation is about the presentation of materials at a high academic level in a way that makes them accessible to all children. There is nothing about the intellectual level of the information that needs simplifying, just the way in which it is presented.

Educationalists, psychologists, parents and policy makers also recognise the need to watch out for indications in behaviour that are signals of distress. The child who closes up is as concerning as the child who plays up. The relationship between stress, dyslexia and giftedness has not been touched upon a great deal in the literature; but the issues are very real.

The question we need to pose therefore is to what extent should we address a child's emotional struggles with the learning process as well as the academic process itself? If children feel alienated from learning they are bound to feel the strain. Policy makers and therefore educationalists often do not seem to value the process of learning, only the achievement of reaching set targets. In such a climate some children are being set up to fail. School is not a voluntary option for them, however hard things get, so there is no way out. The one thing we need to do and so often fail to do through lack of time is to listen to the child and see beyond the behaviour to the cause. However if we are to truly work in a system which values inclusive education for the vast majority of children, we must be aware of specific needs - those which go beyond reaching targets in literacy and numeracy. There is no doubt in my mind that a child's level of intelligence may influence his emotional and behavioural responses to persistent failure, teacher and parent expectations as well as self and peer group expectations.

Despite the level of knowledge that we have these days, there is still a great shortage of training for teachers in the identification, assessment and remediation of gifted dyslexic learners. As a result there can be dire consequences when teachers employ inappropriate attitudes towards such students. There are many gifted learners who whether or not they are dyslexic, have spent years unidentified or mishandled in the classroom. As with dyslexia, inappropriate methods of teaching, low expectations due to apparent poor functioning, bullying in its various forms all lead to immense frustration, low self-esteem and often deviant behaviour.

I personally strongly believe that all children should know what is happening to them, that they are bright, that they have strengths and that there is a reason for their difficulties. So often we have a tendency to speak over the child's head, about them, rather than with them. If we get it right, the sense that they will then have of being heard, understood and valued will often carry them over significant educational and life hurdles.

Whilst we would all agree that the ability to read and write effectively is highly desirable, for some through no fault of their own, despite excellent teaching, it will be difficult to achieve those skills. On the bright side, we must also note that we are entering a new era, that of technology. Computers will read to those who need that level of help, and write upon command for others. The language produced will be appropriate and accurate. For many highly able dyslexic learners, computers may well remove the areas of difficulty leaving them free to develop in the areas in which they perform best – the ideas, the creative and innovative thinking. This in turn will lead to the success that is so rightly theirs alongside high motivation and positive self-esteem.

Conclusion

I believe that the vast majority of gifted dyslexic children are still unidentified in schools today and those few who have been identified are in the main not receiving appropriate provision. There is a great need to highlight the existence of this group and make provision for them at local and national level. The worst thing for them is to place them in classes with under achievers as this is bound to cause severe stress in an already difficult situation. Ideally they should learn in groups with others like themselves so that the 'disability' is put into proportion and the giftedness is highlighted. Specialist teachers need to be fully aware of and trained to deal with their social and emotional needs as well as their academic ones. Raising self-esteem and influencing motivation must be high on the list for training programmes. All gifted learners, dyslexic or not should and could be joining the ranks of the successful. They have the qualities and the ability, if only we could identify them and learn how to nurture them effectively. The uniqueness is there – it is our role to find the way forward.

Useful Reading

1) Meeting the Social and Emotional Needs of Gifted and Talented Children. Michael J. Stopper (Ed.), NACE/Fulton, 2000

2) Dyslexia in Higher Education: policy, provision and practice. The Report of the Working Party on Dyslexia in Higher Education. University of Hull, 1998

3) In the Mind's Eye, West TG, Prometheus Books, 1991

4) Dyslexia: Towards a Better Understanding, Congdon P, Solihull. GCIC, 1981

5) Stress and Dyslexia, Ed: Miles T. and Varma, Whurr, 1995

The Dominie

1 Mandeville Courtyard, 142 Battersea Park Road
London SW11 4NB
Founded in 1987

- A co-educational day school for dyslexic and dyspraxic children between the ages of 6 and 13.

- Whole school approach to remedial education

- 4:1 pupil/staff ratio

- Maximum class size of 8

- CReSTeD registered Category A

For further information and a prospectus please contact:
The Headmistress   020 7720 8783

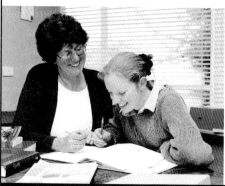

10 Tips for the Numeracy Strategy

It's all very well being presented with big books with in-depth ways of teaching maths to dyslexic individuals, but often just a few quick tips would be helpful. Steve Chinn provides us with a few words of wisdom.

1. Answer basic addition and subtraction facts in two steps, for example to answer 8 + 7, first answer 8 + 8, two eights, to give 16, then take away one to give 15.

2. Do the same with times table facts, again building on the 'easier' facts, working from what the pupil knows. For example to answer 6 x 8 start with 5 x 8 (40) then use 1 x 8 (8), to arrive at 6 x 8 (48). Or answer 4 x 7 as 2 x 7 (14) followed by 2 x 14 (28).

3. For written 'sums' have access to a table square (all the times table facts on a square grid, which will also give the division facts) and an addition square. This removes the problem with remembering the facts and allows the pupil to do and learn the procedures. It should also make work quicker. Speed of working is an issue in maths.

4. Give dyslexic pupils visual, concrete images to support the numbers. For example, illustrate decomposition with coins or base ten blocks. Most, but not all, pupils will benefit from a concrete example which exactly supports the written abstract symbols.

5. Have a basic easy example available as a procedural model. For example, when adding fractions, the most likely mistake is that pupils will add both the top and the bottom numbers as in 1/20 + 1/20 = 2/40 (the correct answer is 2/20). An easy reference example is 1/2 + 1/2 = 2/2 = 1. This also helps in evaluating the answer, "Does it make sense?"

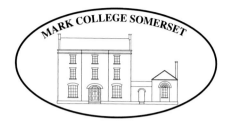

MARK COLLEGE, MARK, SOMERSET TA9 4NP, UK

phone 01278 641 632 or fax 01278 641 426

A secondary school for dyslexic pupils

Mark College is an independent school, approved by the DfEE under section 347 (1) of the Education Act 1996. It is also CReSTeD listed and ISC approved.

Mark College was awarded Beacon School status by the DfEE in September 1999. The College was awarded the Independent Schools Association's Citation of Excellence in 2000.

GCSE results at the College are "outstanding" (Ofsted). This year the percentage of grades at C to A* were 79%. Every Year 11 pupil achieved 7 or more GCSE grades. 75% achieved 5 or more grades at C and above.

Computer facilities are state of the art, with one computer per two boys. This includes two class sets of PC's with voice recognition software and sophisticated and appropriate scanning software.

Sports facilities are first rate, with a full size sports hall, 10 acres of playing fields and two tennis courts. The College pupils achieve great success locally and nationally.

Our Care and boarding arrangements are of "excellent" (Ofsted) standard and achieve top grades in Social Services inspections.

Mathematics teaching at the College is recognised nationally and internationally. "Mathematics for Dyslexics: A Teaching Handbook" written by College Principal, Steve Chinn and College maths teacher, Richard Ashcroft is a standard text. A recent example of the College's innovative work in maths, a CD-Rom "What to do when you can't Learn the Times Tables" was produced in 1999.

A CD-Rom virtual tour of the College is available on request as is the College information Pack

If you have a dyslexic child aged 10 to 14 years, please visit Mark College and see our school at work. Simply phone the College secretary for an appointment.

6. Give back up memory hooks which act as mnemonics. For example all answers to the nine times tables have digits which add up to nine (6 x 9 = 54. 5 + 4 = 9)

7. For word problems encourage the pupil to draw simple pictures to illustrate the problem. For example, the question "Mark is three years older than Jo. If Mark is 11 how old is Jo?" Some pupils will see the word "more" which usually infers add the two numbers, three and eleven, which is wrong in this case. A simple diagram may help to show that Jo is younger than Mark and that you need to subtract.

8. Look carefully at the inconsistencies in the language of time. It is not surprising that dyslexic pupils get confused. We say "Seven ten" and write 7:10, which is in the same order as the words. We say "Ten past seven" and write 7:10, which has the numbers in the opposite order to the words. We say "Ten to seven" and write 6:50, which has neither a 7 nor a 10.

9. As in examples 1 and 2, encourage the pupil to make one hard step into two easy steps. This reduces the time facts have to be held in memory while a calculation is carried out. For example, adding on 9 by counting takes longer than adding 10 and subtracting 1. For example adding £2.99 + £4.99 by adding 9 to 9, carry 1, 9 to 9 plus the carry 1, etc is slow and memory demanding compared to adding £3 and £5 and then subtracting 2p from £8 to give £7.98.

10. Link the processes of mathematics. Learn that addition and subtraction are the same but opposite. Learn that division is done by subtracting in chunks. This clear awareness and understanding sets the foundation for all maths.

APPLEFORD SCHOOL
DfEE & CReSTeD Approved - I.A.P.S. Accredited
Supporting Corporate Member of the British Dyslexia Association

DYSLEXIA
Affects 1 child in 16 mildly - 1 in 25 severely

Appleford School is a co-educational day and boarding school for dyslexic pupils, aged 7 - 13. Pupils are taught the National Curriculum, with particular emphasis on basic literacy and numeracy skills. The whole-school approach at Appleford includes:

* class sizes between 8 - 12 with in-class ancillary support and additional 1 - 1 tutorial support.
* a whole-school approach to dyslexia with research-backed, individual, multisensory programmes, designed to encourage increased self-confidence and self-esteem.
* all teachers are DfEE qualified, with a high ratio of specialist qualifications in dyslexia.
* an extensive games and fixtures programme, numerous challenges and in excess of 30 activities, from claywork to gymnastics, from sewing to judo. A carefully planned and stimulating weekend programme is available.
* a high level of pastoral support geared to the needs of the individual, including weekly PSE sessions.
* experienced, mature and caring houseparents in a friendly, structured boarding situation encouraging the development of personal organisation and life-skills.
* a strong professional support team, including a chartered educational psychologist, speech therapist, occupational therapist and child psychotherapist.

Since Appleford was founded, 84% of our pupils have progressed to such an extent as to enable them to proceed to a mainstream rather than a further specialist school.

Why not visit us, by appointment please, or send for a prospectus?

Appleford School, Shrewton, Salisbury, SP3 4HL
Telephone: 01980 621020   Facsimile: 01980 621366
E-mail: secretary@appleford.demon.co.uk

Assessing learning styles

One of the keys to a successful intervention programme is to discover and harness the learning style of the individual. Here Barbara Given and Gavin Reid review the process.

Controversy over Learning Style

It seems reasonable to assume that the greatest amount of learning can result when teaching is provided to accommodate to a person's learning strengths. This is a common sense assumption and one that is of paramount importance for dyslexic children who may not be able to adapt to a teaching style that focuses on their weaker modalities.

The instruments used to assess learning styles are therefore of great importance. Many critics however attack learning style instruments as lacking in statistical rigour (Curry 1990: Snider 1992) and weak in theoretical definition (Murray-Harvey 1994).

Critics caution that it is difficult to determine how much academic gain results from matching instruction to learning style preferences and how much is due to teacher enthusiasm, novelty and the added focus on how children learn. Experimental studies designed to reduce factors other than instruction matched to style preferences are difficult to implement in authentic classroom settings. Nevertheless experimental research in classrooms does exist - Dunn and colleagues (Dunn et al., 1995) conducted a meta-analysis of 36 experimental research studies from 13 different colleges and studies in the United States. From their review of these studies they concluded that students with strong learning style preferences demonstrated greater academic gains when taught through their preferences than students who had moderate or mixed preferences (Dunn et al., 1995, pg. 358).

Learning Style Approaches

At present there are more than 100 instruments especially designed to identify individual learning styles. Most were developed to evaluate narrow aspects of learning such as preference for visual, auditory, tactile or kinaesthetic input (Grinder 1991). Others are far more elaborate and focus on factors primarily associated with personality issues such as intuition, active experimentation and reflection (Gregorc 1982, 1985; Kolb 1984; Lawrence 1993; Mc Carthy 1987).

Many approaches attempt to identify how individuals process information in terms of its input, memory and expressive functions (Witkin and Goodenough 1981). A few theorists emphasize the body's role in learning and promote cross-lateral movement in hopes of integrating the left and right brain hemispheric activity (Dennison and Dennison 1989). Some perspectives of learning style approaches are briefly described below:

• Riding and Raynor (1998) combine cognitive style with learning strategies. They describe cognitive style as a constraint which includes basic aspects of an individual's psychology such as feeling (affect), doing (behaviour) and knowing (cognition) and the individual's cognitive style relates to how these factors are structured and organised.

• Kolb's (1984) Learning Style Inventory is a derivative of Jung's psychological types combined with Piaget's emphasis on assimilation and accommodation; Lewin's action research model and Dewey's purposeful, experiential learning Kolb's 12-item inventory yields four types of learners: divergers, assimilators, convergers and accommodators.

• The Dunn and Dunn approach (Dunn, Dunn and Price (1996) Learning Styles Inventory contains 104 items that produce a profile of learning style preferences in five domains (environmental, emotional, sociological, physiological and psychological) and 21 elements across those domains. These domains and elements include: environmental (sound, light, temperature, design); emotional (motivation, persistence, responsibility, structure); sociological (learning by self, pairs, peers, team, with an adult), physiological (perceptual preference, food and drink intake, time of day, mobility), and psychological (global or analytic preferences, impulsive and reflective).

• Given (1998) constructed a new model which consists of elements synthesised from other models. This model consists of emotional learning (the need to be motivated by one's own interests), social learning (the need to belong to a compatible group), cognitive learning (the need to know what age-mates know), physical learning (the need to do and be actively involved in learning) and reflective learning (the need to experiment and explore to find what circumstances work best for new learning).

Learning styles using observational criteria

In addition to using standardised instruments, learning styles may be identified to a certain extent through classroom observation. It should be noted that observation in itself may not be sufficient to fully identify learning styles, but the use of a framework for collecting observational data can yield considerable information and can complement the results from more formal assessment.

Observational assessment can be diagnostic, because it is flexible, adaptable and can be used in natural settings with interactive activities. Reid and Given (1999) have developed such a framework – the interactive observational style identification (IOSI). A summary of this is shown below.

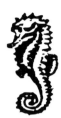

EMOTIONAL

Motivation

- What topics, tasks and activities interest the child?

- What kind of prompting and cueing is necessary to increase motivation?

- What kind of incentives motivate the child – leadership opportunities, working with others, free time or physical activity?

Persistence

- Does the child stick to a task until completion without breaks?

- Are frequent breaks necessary when working on difficult tasks?

Responsibility

- To what extent does the child take responsibility for his/her own learning?

- Does the child attribute success or failure to self or others?

Structure

- Are the child's personal effects (desk, clothing, materials well organised or cluttered?

- How does the child respond to someone imposing organisational structure on him/her?

Social

* Interaction

* When is the child's best work accomplished – when working alone, with one other or in a small group?

* Does the child ask for approval or needs to have work checked frequently?

* Communication.

* Does the child give the main events and gloss over the details?

* Does the child interrupt others when they are talking?

Cognitive

* Modality preference.

* What type of instructions does the child most easily understand - written, oral or visual?

* Does the child respond more quickly and easily to questions about stories heard or read?

* Sequential or simultaneous learning.

* Does the child begin with one step and proceed in an orderly fashion or have difficulty following sequential information?

* Is there a logical sequence to the child's explanations or do her/his thoughts bounce around from one idea to another?

* Impulsive / reflective.

* Are the child's responses rapid and spontaneous or delayed and reflective?

* Does the child seem to consider past events before taking action?

Physical

Mobility

• Does the child move around the class frequently or fidget when seated?

• Does the child like to stand or walk while learning something new?

Food intake

• Does the child snack or chew on a pencil when studying?

Time of day

• During which time of day is the child most alert?

• Is there a noticeable difference between morning work completed and afternoon work?

Reflection

Sound

• Does the child seek out places that are particularly quiet?

Light

• Does the child like to work in dimly lit areas or say that the light is too bright?

Temperature

• Does the child leave his/her coat on when others seem warm?

Furniture Design

• When given a choice does the child sit on the floor, lie down, or sit in a straight chair to read?

Metacognition

• Is the child aware of his/her learning style strengths?

• Does the child demonstrate internal assessment of self by asking questions such as:

• Have I done this before?

• How did I tackle it?

• What did I find easy?

• What was difficult?

• Why did I find it easy or difficult?

• What did I learn?

• What do I have to do to accomplish this task?

• How should I tackle it?

• Should I tackle it the same way as before?

Prediction

• Does the child make plans and work towards goals or let things happen?

Feedback

• How does the child respond to different types of feedback?

• How much external prompting is needed before the child can access previous knowledge?

There are too many manifestations of style to observe all at once. One way to begin the observation process is to select one of the learning systems and progress from there. The insights usually become greater as observation progresses.

Conclusion

It is important to remember that each person possesses five major learning systems that he or she combines in various ways to produce a unique individualised learning style. Without question children as well as adults differ with regard to which system(s) they rely on most for interpreting environmental input and making decisions. Thus, one system may impact how they learn more forcefully than others. Even so, most students learn to work effectively across sensory modalities and across learning systems. By contrast, it is well known that many children with dyslexic difficulties tend to have difficulty shifting from one way of learning to another, and for them it is vitally important that their particular learning style is identified and addressed through teaching that matches how they learn. From this beginning, children can gain confidence in their learning abilities and then explore how others like to learn—in a sense, try something new. Perhaps this experimentation and exploration into what learning conditions work best for them are the most important aspects of a learning-styles curriculum. A thoughtful approach to learning-styles can help find the most effective ways of learning for them. Learning styles instruction, therefore equips children with the skills for life long learning.

References

Curry, Lynn (1990). Learning styles in secondary school: A review of instruments and implications for their use. Ottawa, Ontario, Canada: Curry Adams and Associates, Inc.

Dennison, P. E. & Dennison, G. E. (1989). Brain Gym: Teacher's edition, revised. Ventura, CA: Edu-Kinesthetics, Inc.

Dunn, R., Dunn, K., & Price, G. E. (1975, 1978, 1984, 1987, 1989, 1990, 1996). Learning style inventory. Lawrence, KS: Price Systems.

Dunn, R., Griggs, S., Olson, J., Beasley, M. Gorman, B. (1995). A meta-analytic validation of the Dunn and Dunn model of learning-style preferences. The Journal of Educational Research, 88(61), pp. 353-362.

Given, Barbara (1998). Psychological and neurobiological support for learning-style instruction: Why it works. National Forum of Applied Educational Research Journal, 11(1), 10-15.

Given, B K and Reid, G (1998) The Interactive Observation Style Identification, Personal Correspondence

Given, B.K. and Reid, G. (1999) Learning Styles, A Guide for Teachers and Parents. Red Rose Publications, 22 St. Georges Road, St.Annes on Sea, Lancashire, FY8 2AE

Gregorc, Diane F. (1997). Relating to style. Columbia, CT: Gregorc Associates, Inc.

Grinder, Michael. (1991). Righting the educational conveyor belt (2nd ed.). Portland, OR: Metamorphous Press.

Kolb, David (1984). Experiential learning: Experience as the source of learning and development. Englewood Cliffs, NJ: Prentice-Hall, Inc.

Lawrence, Gordon (1979/1982/1993). People types and tiger stripes (3rd ed.). Gainsville, FL: Center for Applications of Psychological Type, Inc.

McCarthy, Bernice (1980/1987). The 4mat system: Teaching to learning styles with right/left mode techniques. Barrington, IL:

Murray-Harvey, Rosalind (1994). Conceptual and measurement properties of the productivity environmental preference survey as a measure of learning style. Educational and Psychological Measurement, 54(4), pp. 1002-1012.

Riding, R. and Rayner, S. (1998) Cognitive Styles and Learning Strategies, Understanding Style Differences in Learning and Behaviour, David Fulton Publishers, London

Witkin, Herman and Goodenough, Donald (1981). Cognitive styles: Essence and origins. Psychological Issues Monograph 51. New York: International Universities Press.

Dr. Barbara Given is an Associate Professor at George Mason University, Virginia, USA and Dr. Gavin Reid is a Senior Lecturer at the University of Edinburgh.

DYSLEXIA:
At the dawn of the new century
18–21 April 2001

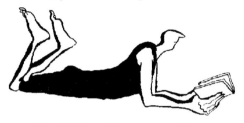

Special Section - Whole School Approach

Every subject is different - or is it?

In this Special Section on a Whole School Approach, Neil Mackay, a dyslexia consultant in north Wales, ask subject teachers how they contribute to the effective whole school strategy.

St David's College, Llandudno

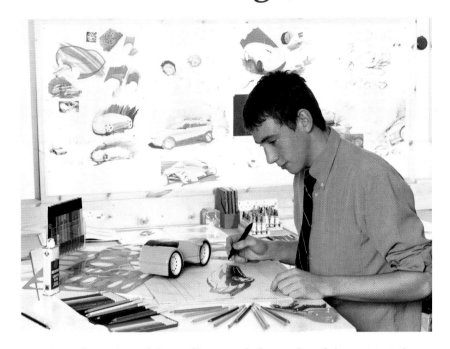

Co-educational boarding and day school (age 11–18)

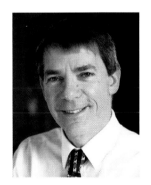

"Our whole school approach to dyslexia extends beyond the classroom into a wide range of sports, hobbies and outdoor pursuits – all aimed at building up the self-belief and confidence of the boys and girls who join us. We have 35 years' successful experience at developing strategies to support dyslexic pupils and pride ourselves on tailoring our curriculum to the individual. We have particularly strong facilities for encouraging design skills through Art, Design & Technology and Computer Aided Design.

If you would like to know more, please telephone my secretary, Mrs Sue Hold, on 01492 875974."

William Seymour

William Seymour M.A. - Headmaster

St David's College, Llandudno, North Wales LL30 1RD

St. David's College is a registered charity providing a whole-person education within a Christian framework.

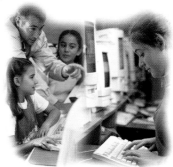
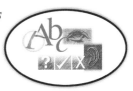

Introduction

Many parents of dyslexic children dread the thought of the move to a secondary school; the sheer size and number of teachers seems to intimidate the parents more than it does their children! It needs to be appreciated that secondary schools are set up to operate as a big institution and deliberately use the pastoral system to break the units down into manageable sizes. In most schools the unit is the year group, often with about 180 pupils and 6 –8 form teachers, supported by a Head of Year and overseen by a senior manager. In fact this unit is about the size of many primary schools and can work extremely well on behalf of dyslexic pupils.

Parents choosing a secondary school are right to consider the specialist qualifications of the SENCo. However it is important to realise that most children will meet at least eight subject teachers each week, and the "dyslexia friendliness" of a school rests very much on the shoulders of the non-dyslexia specialist subject teachers.

The contributors to this chapter are, with one exception, subject teachers in secondary schools. They teach across the ability range, often including A level classes, and have considerable experience at making the curriculum work for dyslexic pupils. Their articles reflect not only their subject expertise, which is essential at GCSE, but their understanding of how children learn and their willingness to do what is necessary, in terms of materials and learning styles, to make sure that everyone in the class is learning. One contributor, whose school invests heavily to ensure that all pupils are supported to interact with text in an ability appropriate way, also highlights the importance of study skills. Some of the contributors work at a school which achieved 5+ A-G passes for each Year 11 pupil in the recent GCSE exams, a 100%

success rate which suggests that they must be doing something right!

The contributor who is not a subject teacher, Elizabeth Turner, runs an LEA funded Dyslexia Resource within a large and very successful secondary school. A published author in her own right, being the co-author of a book on dyslexia, her article discusses the importance of specialist teachers being a positive role model and contributing to the life of the whole school.

The Role of a Dyslexia Resource Teacher in a Comprehensive Secondary School

Elizabeth Turner is the teacher in charge of Dyslexia Resource at Hawarden High School, Flintshire, North Wales.

Background

Hawarden High School in Flintshire, North Wales was designated and specifically resourced for severely dyslexic pupils in September 1992 as a County provision. The Resource, which is now in its ninth year of operation, caters for up to fifteen pupils within a framework of a whole school approach to Dyslexia and a dyslexia friendly environment. It also offers Sixth form support. The needs of pupils with statements, whose Resource placement has been allocated by County in liaison with the school, are therefore the shared responsibility of all the staff. The role of the specialist teacher attached to the school and working within the Resource is primarily to lead and co-ordinate that responsibility and to provide specific learning support for the Resource pupils. The role in managing, teaching and leading the Resource is therefore diverse.

Teaching Role

The funding for the full time Resource Teacher is met by the LEA, which also provides funding for a full time classroom assistant, secretarial support and resource capitation. Admission to the Resource is via the County SEN Co-Ordinator in consultation with the school and moderation panel. There are County criteria in place for admission purposes. The Secretary of State (or Appeals Tribunal) may also decide on placement providing there is a vacancy.

Curriculum provision is based on pupils' needs and there is appropriate disapplication from National Curriculum in order to deliver the programmes of study that are designed to help overcome the dyslexic difficulties. At Hawarden this involves disapplication from modern foreign languages. Parents are notified of this before they accept a placement and their agreement required. If a pupil is gifted linguistically there is provision/ opportunity/ flexibility built into the system to allow that pupil to pick up German in Year 9 if appropriate.

In Years 7 - 9 pupils receive 5 hours per week (1 hour daily) tuition in the Resource on a pupil teacher ratio of 3:1. The emphasis is on multisensory teaching, the core of which is a phonic/spelling and reading programme. Running alongside this is the study skills element, access to age appropriate literature and counselling in managing the literacy difficulty.

In years 10 and 11 Resource time is reduced to 2.5 hours per week recognising the demands, pressures and stress the GCSE examinations, coursework and curriculum have on the dyslexic pupil. The time is tutorial based and pupils are encouraged to bring their own work from curriculum areas with them at this time. Study skills are continued using a scaffolding approach with the pupil's own work being the impetus. This makes the tasks more meaningful and helpful to the pupil and prevents overloading. The phonic programme is not used at this stage but learning strategies using a multisensory approach are continued as well as techniques for revision and examinations. Counselling in managing the literacy difficulties continues and careers support advice is given at this time.

Tutorial periods are vital in Years 10 and 11. Thomson and Watkins (1991) strongly recommend that time is given over for this purpose in the last two years of compulsory schooling.

This is because a window of opportunity exists when an informal approach can work to good effect. The message is that the teacher has time to support the individual and can relieve some of the mounting pressures that loom ahead with external examinations. Tutorial time is also useful for the revisiting and revising of areas of uncertainty as well as the rewording of explanations and clarification of ideas. The individual can sort out academic problems as well as unloading the personal, social and emotional issues which many dyslexics carry around with them.

Assessment Role

The assessment role of the Resource teacher is varied. It involves the supervising and administration of appropriate tests and continuous assessment as part of a comprehensive monitoring process, the evaluating of the 'value added factor', the identification of strengths and weaknesses in the curriculum in relation to a pupil's specific learning differences, the assessing of learning needs and styles of a pupil at Key Stage 3 and 4 and transferring that information to curriculum areas.

This is a two way process. It allows learning to be transferred across the curriculum and prevents the work of the Resource being seen by Staff, parents and pupils as a separate entity. It helps to overcome what a pupil was heard to comment in the early days of the Resource's existence:

"You go to extra English in that little room with that Lady! Is she a real teacher?"

It is very important that the Resource teacher is not seen as 'special' but is regarded and seen as another teacher in the school. The Resource teacher should not stand out as 'odd' in appearance or manner but conform loosely to what the

Fairley House School

30 Causton Street London SW1P 4AU

Telephone 020 7976 5456 Fax: 020 7976 5905
Principal Mrs Jacqueline Ferman BA, MEd
E-mail: office@fairleyhouse.westminster.sch.uk

Status: Independent DfEE registered 427/6327
Age range: 6 - 12
Number on Roll: 95
24 teaching staff/therapists
4 teaching assistants
Type: Coed, Day

Special needs catered for: Specific learning difficulties (dyslexia and dyspraxia). This can include problems with receptive and expressive language, with information processing, with auditory and visual recall and with fine and gross motor control. Entrants must be of at least average intelligence without significant physical or behavioural problems and must have English as a first language. Up to one third of the children are financed by a local authority.

Specialist facilities: The National Curriculum is taught, with emphasis on information technology and word processing. The teaching style is modified and the content adapted so that every lesson is accessible to every child. Daily intensive special provision is provided in basic numeracy and literacy in small groups. Each child receives individual special provision tuition. The multi-disciplinary team includes 2 full-time speech and language and 2 occupational therapists on site. An educational psychologist spends 1 day a week in school.

Home/School links: Parents are counselled at the initial assessment of the child, and thereafter provided with ongoing support, especially prior to the child's transfer to the next school. There are termly reports, parent/teacher meetings and access at other times. Lectures and social functions are held regularly. Homework is closely monitored.

General Environment: The architecturally designed premises are light and spacious. The Assembly Hall has a stage for theatrical and musical productions. There are separate, fully-equipped rooms for the School Library, Design Technology, Science, Computing and Music. There is a playground opposite and local facilities for games and swimming. The school's location in central London allows visits to museums and to other places of interest.

teenager expects teachers to be. A teenager usually wants to belong to a peer group and the Resource teacher should also conform to the 'peer groups' of other teachers. How many emerging adolescents have asked parents what they are wearing etc for parents evening - not wanting their mother / father/ guardian to stand out from the crowd in some outlandish apparel. It is the same with the Resource teacher - being special means being normal and blending in. The cringe factor can easily come into force here - this is inclusion in its fullest sense!

One of the main purposes of assessment is formative: to provide information to help people make decisions. Effective assessment has clear purposes that make planning more effective and shapes the future learning of the pupil. It should enhance teacher skills, promote continuity and make demands for greater accountability. Assessment is not an end in itself but a means of arriving at a better understanding of a child's learning difficulties, remembering that it is the important that must be made measurable, not the measurable important.

Pastoral Role

When a dyslexic pupil enters the secondary phase there is usually a period of adjustment. This can be due to a variety of reasons from being in an environment away from home/catchment area and friends to the adjustment which many pupils have to face in moving from a small primary to a large comprehensive school. Hopefully the majority of pupils adapt swiftly but there is sometimes a small minority that may take longer than expected. They have poor self image and need support and counselling at this time to adapt to the challenge. One of the main reasons for their apparent unhappiness is that they have been removed from friends at previous schools and feel isolated. Another reason for these negative feelings is a fear of failure itself. Many severely dyslexic pupils are skilled at failure having been exposed to it on a daily basis for a number of years. To bring about a change of attitude in themselves and to minimize their fear of trying in case they fail, the Resource teacher needs to counsel them on managing the literacy difficulties and fully explain, often explicitly, the nature of dyslexia itself, pointing out strengths and weaknesses and emphasizing the positive advantages of being dyslexic.

Supportive Role

Support for learning has different aspects and outcomes. Supporting colleagues with suggestions and techniques for working with dyslexic pupils is one important aspect of support and supporting the curriculum itself through differentiation and modification is another. Although all pupils have entitlement to the curriculum, without access this is meaningless.

Liaison Role

One of the fundamental principles of the Code of Practice is that partnership with parents is essential. For the Resource teacher this partnership is crucial - it is a tripartite relationship between home, school and the pupil. Liaison never means confrontation but participation, understanding and support.

Management and Organisation

The managerial role of the Resource teacher involves many aspects of administration. There is the actual setting up of policy, practice and procedure in running a Resource. There is the ordering of equipment, books and audio visual necessities. There is the writing of the cross curricula IEPs, the monitoring of progress as well as the writing of the specific programmes of work. Liaising with Year heads, Form tutors, Faculty Heads, individual teachers and outside agencies are all part of the day-to-day management role.

Staff Development/ Inset

An important part of the role of a Dyslexia Resource teacher is to heighten awareness of Dyslexia itself. It is essentially spreading the word and sharing good practice. This is done by a variety of means. The Resource is open to visitors on request, from in and out of County and also from other countries. The Resource Teacher provides Inset on dyslexia for the County to teachers from Key Stages 3 and 4. Topics covered are on the varied aspects of dyslexia and range from spelling, reading, handwriting, mindmapping and resources for dyslexia, to multisensory learning and memory .

The role of a Dyslexia Resource teacher is not straightforward and simple but diverse and many layered. The most obvious part of the role is the teaching one but there are other equally responsible strands to the role. They all play their part in the whole package. They are all essential components because what is being dealt with here is the whole child.

Bibliography

Payne, T. and Turner, E. 1999. Dyslexia, A Parents' and Teachers' Guide, Multilingual Matters Ltd

Pollock, J Waller, E.1994. Day- to -Day Dyslexia in the Classroom, Routledge

Thomson, ME and Watkins, EJ.1991 Dyslexia : A Teaching Handbook, Whurr Publishers

Things to Think About When Teaching English Literature to Dyslexic Pupils.

Jayne Pughe is SENCo at Hawarden High School, Flintshire, North Wales.

These basic strategies are part of all my teaching. Teaching dyslexic pupils makes you think a little harder about your approaches but they do not create an extra preparation 'burden' because these approaches just enable all pupils to access literature. Good special needs practice is good teaching practice.

Teaching the language of literature.

At the start of the GCSE course there is a whole English Literature vocabulary that has to be explicitly taught. This offers an opportunity to introduce subject specific language and remind pupils of coping strategies for spelling. The difficulty of unfamiliar language provides a non-patronising framework to teach syllables, mnemonics, memory aids and spelling rules.

A worthwhile exercise is getting pupils to make a poster that represents their strategy for remembering a new word. The language that is needed in Literature essays is therefore represented in their environment, as are useful spelling strategies.

Oracy

The usefulness of oral work as preparation for written literature tasks cannot be over emphasised. In literature, exploration of character, plot, theme and atmosphere are essential skills. Pupils are able to do this more successfully if they have been allowed to discuss their ideas in informal or formal situations. Also drama activities develop empathy and a deeper moral understanding of a piece of literature.

Oral planning is beneficial for many reasons. Pupils are willing to invest time and energy into planning a task because they are talking; this doesn't threaten their confidence like writing. As they have invested in their planning and received positive feedback from their teacher and peers they feel a sense of ownership of the work. I have seen pupils attack essays with vigour because their planning has been so successful.

How to reinforce learning

When pupils reach Year Ten it is easy to take certain things for granted. I used to assume that pupils suddenly learnt to organise their revision notes even though I knew that I hadn't until I was at college. Pupils need to be explicitly taught how to use colour coding, pictures, spider diagrams, mnemonics etc. They then need to be encouraged to experiment with these techniques and to jettison the ones that do not suit their learning style. They also need to be taught how to annotate texts and handouts. They need help with the organisation of their handouts. A session spent organising notes can be useful if it shows any gaps in teaching or in an individual's notes.

Notes given in class and tasks will be more helpful if the skills they demand are varied. If we access a text through many channels: listening, reading, viewing, reasoning, prediction, empathy and physical tasks everybody's strongest learning style will be catered for. This was made clear to me when a pupil felt that a mapping exercise based on Stone Cold helped her to understand the split narrative and appreciate the tension.

Planning and drafting

Again these are skills that must be explicitly taught to GCSE pupils. The provision of a scaffold is essential for pieces of coursework but pupils must be taught how to produce their own scaffolds. Modelling good practice is a useful exercise. Looking at successful pieces of coursework from a previous year on a different text and deciding what each paragraph consists of can be a starting point. Then the class can produce a group scaffold for their own text.

An extremely helpful task is also to look at examination style questions and plan answers for homework on a regular basis. Sharing these plans reinforces the skill for those who are successful but also again provides extra modelling for those who are still developing their ability to plan.

Finding quotations that reinforce certain points is another crucial part of the planning process. This can be an extremely daunting task and therefore when preparing coursework group 'searches' can eliminate a great deal of stress. Make sure that pupils look for a number of alternatives for each point and encourage debate about who has the stronger quotation. This will ensure that pupils develop an interest in dissecting literature and this also fosters the idea that many alternative interpretations are valid in this subject area.

Drafting is always an extremely difficult thing to approach especially when a pupil has invested a great deal of time into a first draft. If pupils provide their own framework for re-drafting they always want to improve the spelling and the handwriting. Making sure that pupils are aware of the Literature marking criteria provides a helpful stimulus for re-drafting. By offering the criteria in more concrete and accessible terms it is possible to help pupils to look at their work and the work of their peers in order to set achievable and relevant targets for improvement.

Dyslexia in Science

Dr Graham Simpkin, Ysgol John Bright, Llandudno and Sue Simpkin Hawarden High School, Flintshire, North Wales. Both are science teachers.

Science is a subject where dyslexic students will be affected by all the same problems that they encounter in other subjects because, although science is a practical subject there is still a reliance on the written word in both presenting information and assessing work.

There are a number of issues that will pose particular problems within science lessons – the spelling of scientific words, coping with complex instructions, organising and sequencing work - are some of the problems experienced.

Spelling problems within science – many words in science do not follow the spelling rules that can help students in other areas of use of English, such as the 'i' before 'e' rule, many scientific words are derived from Greek and this rule does not apply, including the word 'science' itself. This particular problem with spelling can undermine the student who can cope with the science. It is acceptable for a student to spell words as they sound using phonics though this may not be as acceptable to parents. In science, throughout key stages 3 and 4, there are many long technical words that have to be split up into syllables to aid spelling as would happen in other areas.

A successful strategy is to use a subject specific dictionary. This can be tailored to the specific strengths and learning strategies of the student. Technical words can be recorded as phonics with conventional spellings alongside, or diagrams with spellings.

Following complex instructions – within practical lessons the teacher often gives a series of instructions that have to be followed in sequence if the experiment is to be a success. This can be a problem for a number of students but can be a particular problem for dyslexic students.

The consequence of this is that in many experiments as in cookery the method has to be followed in the correct order or the experiment may not do what the teacher expects or may not do anything at all. The first of these can be irritating but the experiment failing to work can be very discouraging for all.

There are a number of strategies that can help in this situation. The particular approach will depend on the strengths of the particular student.

All students will cope better with a process that has been itemised into a number of individual steps. This can be extended for those that have a good concept of number – by numbering the steps. Some students will find the process easier if the steps are portrayed diagrammatically. Putting the steps of the process onto individual cards, which have to be sorted initially, is an alternative method of itemising the steps.

The need to work in pairs in most practical situations can work to the advantage of the science teacher coping with dyslexic students within a large class. Judicial pairing to form the groups can aid the dyslexic student who can draw on the strengths of the partner.

Linked with the problem of complex instructions is the more general problem of organisation of work in class and organisation of written reports – this is a particular problem when working towards coursework in KS 3 and 4.

Many dyslexic students can carry out the practical aspects of the science curriculum only to fall behind when recording their work to allow for assessment. The problem is that we are still largely reliant on the written record of work completed.

Those with very weak writing skills should be encouraged to

record their work orally but there is still the problem of ordering the record to provide a logical account.

The use of prepared frameworks or templates with headings can help to organise accounts. The use of 'postits' to record the various parts of the work will allow the work to be ordered before a final 'hard copy' is made.

With the bright dyslexic student the final written task may be expected to be completed at home which will pose problems of the verification of authenticity when work is eventually presented.

A final problem in science arises with the majority of textbooks. Modern textbooks are well structured with short sentences but this means that each sentence can be a vital fact written in technical language making hard work for the dyslexic student. This is a problem that cannot be easily avoided except by producing student specific worksheets.

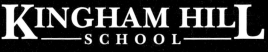
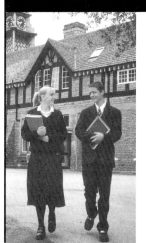

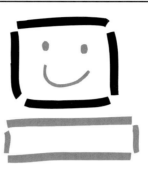

Touch-type, Read & Spell

COMPUTER COURSE

A multi-sensory - hearing, speaking, touching - computer aided learning course based on the textbook

Alpha to Omega

ALPHA TO OMEGA IS WRITTEN BY BEVÉ HORNSBY, FRULA SHEAR AND JULIE POOL

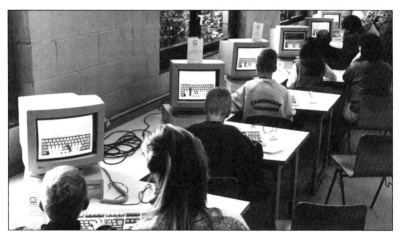

Spelling and Reading Development through Touch-typing
School licences, Local Education Authority contracts,
private centres and supported Home CD-Rom Course.
For further details please contact Philip Alexandre MA, DPSE, Cert Ed.
National Course Director, PO Box 535, Bromley, Kent BR1 2YF
Tel: 020 8464 1330   Fax: 020 8313 9454

History and the Dyslexic Child

Jim Roberts, Head of History at Hawarden High School, Flintshire, North Wales.

According to the National Curriculum for Wales all pupils at Key Stage 3 should be:

"Given opportunities to build on the knowledge, understanding and skills acquired at Key Stage 2. In addition, these pupils should in chronological order, know about the main political, economic, social and cultural features of selected periods from the histories of Wales and Britain."

Therefore, each pupil will have to show an awareness of the following Historical Skills:

- Chronological awareness

- Historical knowledge and understanding

- Interpretation of history

- Historical enquiry

- Organisation and communication

These five areas make up the study of History, and for the dyslexic student can be very difficult concepts and ideas to come to terms with. I will try to deal with the approaches that are taken towards the teaching of chronology and historical enquiry and organisation and communication; these are perhaps the most difficult areas for dyslexic students.

Chronological Awareness

For the History teacher, telling the story of events is perhaps the easiest aspect of the subject; however, the story has to be set in its correct chronological sequence. This is where many dyslexic students find difficulty in sorting out the concept of time.

As Payne and Turner point out:

"History might present difficulties for a dyslexic when faced with chronology and the identification of historical events in relation to time. Matching an historical event to a specific date is a similar activity to matching a sound with a symbol."

In Hawarden, the understanding of chronology is one of the first skills all students must learn although this concept is something with which they are supposed to be familiar. Many students whether dyslexic or not find the concept of time difficult to understand. In Hawarden, the approach that we take is to use timelines. A timeline is a line drawn to a specific scale to represent a period. Normally there are three stages in the building up of timelines for students

- A timeline with scale 1cm equals one-year, which is drawn to a length of 12cm and important events of the student's life are marked on it.

- Secondly a timeline with a scale 1cm equals ten years, which is drawn to a length of 10cm which is the measurement of a century. Normally, important events from the 20th century are placed on this as well as the student's year of birth. This helps to give the student the idea that time is vast.

- Thirdly a timeline with a scale 1cm equals a hundred years which is drawn to a length of 23cms. On this line is marked the student's year of birth as well as significant events from the past. The hope is that students will be able to visualise the past and be able to see something which is an intangible.

The working out of the length of a reign, an era or dynasty are crucial to the development of chronological awareness. These words are historical jargon words from which there is no escape. However, if students realise that these are just another way of describing periods, then they understand even more the need for dates.

However, the teaching of the concept of time necessitates the teaching of AD and BC. The teaching of a degree of numeracy is inescapable when dealing with time. For most students they are able to understand for AD that it is necessary to add on to a date to work out the length of a reign. For example "Elizabeth 1 came to the throne in 1558 and ruled for 45 years. When did her reign end?"

The concept of BC is by far the most difficult concept for many students to come to terms with, however there is a simple rule that is applied in school when dealing the concept of BC. This is the idea of backward counting i.e. counting back down to zero. For example, if a man or woman is born in 100BC and lives for 50 years, what is the year of his death? Students would hopefully realise from the letters BC that they must take away 50 from 100 to arrive at the answer: 50BC. Or if they are in difficulty use their timeline to work out the problem.

Historical Inquiry

Historical inquiry requires students to have high order reading skills if they are to cope with the sources of historical evidence. There is a debate within history over how much modification should be made to the sources to make them more accessible. The problem is that if sources are modified too much then they are no longer historical sources. The jargon words such as primary and secondary sources are explained below:

- Primary Sources are something from the time an event happened.

- Secondary sources are pieces of information written about events much later, e.g. a school textbook. These definitions are placed in the student's History Dictionary where all jargon words are kept.

Then the students begin to examine simple sources working out whether they are primary or secondary. This is normally undertaken in groups where they decide why a source is primary or secondary and give a reason. All groups answer before the correct answer is given and then we examine as a group why some gave wrong answers. The approach that is taken in Hawarden is to make the sources as manageable as possible by breaking them up into sentences and as a group reading the sentence together. When a comparison of sources is to be made, the idea is to spot the difference or deliberate mistake. Teachers will carefully examine one source with the group and extrapolate a list of five or more points which the students will have with them. Next the second source will be given, read together line by line. The students will be asked to find a number of differences; the first one is normally completed for them. In many cases, clues or guides will be given to the students to make the task more accessible. The majority of students find this activity enjoyable and it enables them to use sources without making the reading too onerous and giving them a sense of achievement. As their skill level develops increasingly demanding sources and tasks can be built into their work.

Organisation and communication

Related to the use of sources is Organisation and Communication of written work. This is the most problematic area for many dyslexic students so basic rules are given:

- Make sure your work has a title and is dated.

• Write in sentences.

• Check the spelling of historical terms.

• Make sure you can read what you have written.

• Correct any mistakes immediately.

These instructions are followed by exercises such as filling in the missing words, using poster diagrams to transmit the historical concept and by role-play. Role-play is one of the most effective ways of communicating difficult ideas. For example, a group of students played the characters of individuals involved in the Norman Conquest. Then they were asked to explain who they were and why they wanted to be King of England. Also, the others had to decide who they then thought had the best claim to the throne, a difficult concept of cause and consequence which was easily understood because of the role-play activity.

Written work is set, following the rules that the students are given. In most cases, they are given writing frames. Specific targets for the number of sentences that they have to write on topics, which include key words or phrases, are also given.

History is a difficult subject but it is accessible for all students and dyslexic students actually find history rewarding as they can find a wide range of material using ICT as well as videos and the traditional textbook.

Planning and organisation: the key to success in PE/Games

Harold Abrams is Head of Physical Studies, Ysgol Bro Llyn

Read the SEN Register

Many PE teachers believe that their subject offers failing pupils a chance to excel and, in consequence, some prefer to "take children as they find them" rather than build in preconceptions formed through reading the opinions of others. Admirable though this may be in principle, in practice it can mean setting a child up to fail through not being forewarned.

Knowing who is dyslexic, empowers PE teachers to anticipate needs and to meet them before they arise.

Getting Changed

This can be a nightmare for pupils, teachers and parents alike! The rush to get out of uniform and into kit can often mean that shoes, socks, ties etc find their way to the furthest flung corners of the changing room. When it is time to get changed back the teacher may be met with accusations of theft/mischief or, as the changing room empties, a bemused and tearful child searching under benches for articles of clothing.

Having identified dyslexic pupils via the SEN Register the teacher is able to:

- Plan lessons to allow extra changing time at the beginning and end.

- Check that trainer/boot laces are tied and offer discreet help as pupils leave the changing room; asking dyslexic pupils to drop into the PE office on the way out is one way.

- Stipulate a "changing procedure" for all - require that, for example, ties are placed in trouser/skirt pockets and socks in shoes, trousers/skirts are always hung on a peg with shirt/blouse over the top. Also it is worth demanding that kit is put back into bags as it is taken off.

- Repeat the check before pupils leave for the next lesson

- Supervise the changing for a few weeks, offering help as appropriate and personally organising the search for missing clothing with charm and good humour.

The Big Picture

A lesson introduction which answers the five basic questions:

- Who?
- What?
- Why?
- Where?
- When?

in whatever order matches the task, gives all pupils an overview of what is required, something dyslexic youngsters find particularly helpful.

Buddy Time

"Buddy time" is structured opportunities for oracy, when groups discuss and plan their sequence, strategy, tactics, dance moves etc. By building in a report back procedure it is also possible to confirm that instructions are understood and the task is proceeding as planned.

On-Task Monitoring

Despite all of the good practice outlined above, profound short term memory issues often associated with dyslexia may still make it difficult for instructions to be followed. It is good practice, therefore, to keep a special eye on dyslexic pupils to make sure that they are on-task and that their work is proceeding appropriately. The following phrases may be helpful:

• "Just remind me what you have done so far/have to do next."

• "Explain to your partner/group what you have to do next. Is this right?"

Recording

The recording of times, scores etc is an essential part of many lessons, but not a task that should be allocated to a dyslexic pupil without due consideration. Once again, a thorough knowledge of the pupils on the SEN Register will prevent someone being "set up to fail". This is not to say that dyslexic youngsters cannot or should not be expected to take their share of recording tasks. However more time will be needed and some "buddy" backup will be advantageous.

Developing Motor Skills

Some dyslexic youngsters lack certain fine and gross motor skills - they may be dyspraxic, clumsy or whatever. PE has an opportunity to contribute to the neurological development of dyslexic children, particularly those with a somewhat immature central nervous system. In particular, teachers can pay their pupils the compliment of never giving up: if it is important that certain physical skills are learnt then dyslexic youngsters deserve the opportunity for over-learning in a structured way.

Just as adult non-readers have been made to crawl as part of their reading lessons, the development of the central nervous system that comes with learning and consolidating new motor skills can only be of benefit.

Hot Tips for science

Sion O'Neil is science teacher at Bryn Teg High School, Anglesey

Aims, Goals and Objectives

A statement of aims, goals and objectives at the start of each lesson helps dyslexic learners put the activity in context. In particular it makes very clear what is required, how it will be achieved and what will be marked. Many youngsters find it easier to minimise short term memory problems when they have the big picture.

Jargon Words

Science is littered with complicated, polysyllabic jargon words which need to be correctly spelt. In-house science dictionaries are very successful, as are key words pasted around the walls. The best way to support dyslexic youngsters to learn jargon words is to use letter tiles ("Scrabble" letters are ideal) to harness the power of multi-sensory learning. This method works well as a "buddy" activity and operates like this:

- Give a pupil the jumbled letters which make up a jargon word.

- Ask the pupil to make the word, saying the letter names as s/he puts the letters together.

- Jumble and repeat.

- When this is firm, repeat stages 2 and 3 but this time requiring the pupil to select the letters from the bag/box.

Time invested in this procedure is money in the bank later on, especially at Key Stage 4.

Following Instructions

Much of Science is sequential and it is important that stages are gone through in a particular order. Although many dyslexic youngsters have a talent for science, sequencing is not always a strength! Sequential memory issues can be minimised in a multi-sensory way:

- Cards or laminated pages headed "Equipment", "Method", etc can be made available as an aide memoir.

- "Post-its" can be used to write up the appropriate section and then stuck onto the headed card, to be written up, in order, at the end of the experiment.

- Experiment instructions can be cut into strips to be re-ordered - this is very effective and seems to benefit a majority of pupils.

On-Task Monitoring

Despite all of the good practice outlined above, profound short term memory issues often associated with dyslexia may still make it difficult for instructions to be followed. It is good practice, therefore, to keep a special eye on dyslexic pupils to make sure that they are on-task and that their work is proceeding appropriately. The following phrases may be helpful:

- "Just remind me what you have done so far/have to do next."

- "Explain to your partner/group what you have to do next. Is this right?"

Calculations and Recording

Problems with the stages of long multiplication and/or division may cause a dyslexic pupil, who has performed the experiment to perfection, to make a mess of the results and hence the conclusion. There can be no substitute for "management by walking about" at this stage, the dyslexia friendly science teacher taking the opportunity to look over shoulders and intervene as appropriate.

Recording neatly and in a way in which the information can be used later is often a problem for dyslexic youngsters. Pre-printed proformas and skeleton tables containing some headings and/or some of the information with the rest to be inserted by the pupil are two ways of minimising recording problems.

The accurate recording of homework is often an issue and can be compounded by a poorly presented set of results. The potentially unpopular bottom line is that, if the child is identified as dyslexic in the SEN Register, it is the responsibility of the teacher to ensure that homework is properly recorded and that all relevant data is available and legible.

Write Ups

Science write ups lend themselves to the "framework" approach, in which each section takes the form of a pre-headed box. It is often helpful to include a paragraph starter at the top of each box as a lead in e.g.

METHOD

First we had to.........

Then we.........

After that.....

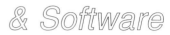
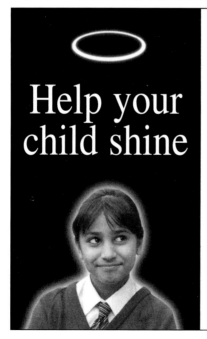

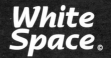

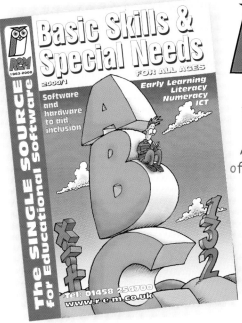
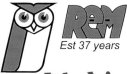

On targets with DARTS

Neil Gibbons is Deputy Headteacher at St. Richard Gwyn High School in Flintshire.

I wanted to call the course DARTS (Directed Activities Related to Text) after the 1979 Schools Council project on the effective use of reading but I realised that this might be open to misinterpretation! "Secondary pupils waste curriculum time playing darts" was not the title we wanted. So the course was given the more neutral title of "Skills" when it was introduced in 1994.

Skills is not a remedial programme for particular pupils; it is a language based programme of work for all year 7 pupils. Each mixed ability class has one lesson of Skills each week on their timetable. The course lasts the whole year (approximately 38 hours of instruction) and aims to foster reading as a thinking activity.

We believe that language development is stimulated particularly by techniques which focus the reader's attention on the text at the word, phrase, sentence or paragraph level. The development of these skills requires a structured programme of activities which accommodates the differing levels of reading competence achieved by pupils during the previous key stage. The activities include:

- **Cloze Procedure**

This is an effective means of teaching the use of context cues and anticipation skills.

- **Sequencing**

This encourages readers to make use of semantic and syntactic cues when deciding on a logical sequence for the segments of text.

• Prediction

This requires careful reading of the text and calls upon a number of important skills, especially the higher order skill, inference.

• Modelling

Pupils are required to restructure what they have read, perhaps in the form of a diagram, graph, drawing etc.

• Writing Frameworks

These help pupils to extend their written responses by providing a structure on which to build.

• Responding to questions

Pupils are encouraged to develop their own skills of argument and reasoning, helped by verbal and pictorial stimulus.

The activities are designed to enable each child to respond in a way that will result in the successful completion of each task at an ability appropriate level. Although some commercially available material is used a lot of "in-house" activities have been devised because there is no one scheme flexible enough to achieve the aims of the course. Also many of the schemes on the market are incredibly dry, containing little but dull worksheets.

We use unwanted photographs which are presented as mini jigsaws to be completed before we move on to doing the same with "bits of text." Christmas cards are also cut into progressively smaller pieces and reassembled as the pupil tries to remember the original picture. I particularly enjoy feigning a sneezing attack at the crucial moment! We then discuss the importance of visual cues when trying to understand a new passage.

The organisation of the lessons and the pattern of classroom grouping will depend on the work being undertaken. Sometimes pupils will work individually, sometimes in friendship groups and sometimes in groups dictated by the teacher. Also pupils will be working at different attainment levels and using different materials within the scheme. Of course this does not mean that pupils are physically grouped according to ability, but it is important that reading tasks are challenging at an appropriate level of ability. This means that assessment is important and all pupils take the Cognitive Abilities Test (CATs) as part of their Skills lesson in the first term. The profile is shared with colleagues and with parents and, most importantly, is used to plan the programme of work for the individual.

Although I teach in the English department it is not expected that the Skills lessons are taught by English staff. Originally I taught all the classes (very useful for a senior member of staff with responsibility for curriculum and assessment!) but timetable constraints meant that staff from other departments had to become involved. This has had many benefits; not only do those staff have a better understanding of the aims of the language development course, but some of them have actually enjoyed teaching a "subject" outside of the National Curriculum. Ideas and approaches are taken back into other subject areas and the course itself benefits from fresh approaches.

There are disadvantages as well, particularly in terms of transferability of skills. Pupils do tend to forget the skills they have learnt, especially when these are not further developed in the context of other lessons. Obviously I would like more time on the curriculum, but then so would every other teacher. Given the time I would like to run a timetabled course for pupils in Year 10 to develop appropriate support strategies for GCSE.

I have deliberately not mentioned pupils with dyslexia yet. The course is not designed for a particular group of pupils, but it does fit in with our overall philosophy of being open about pupils who experience language difficulties. More than this, we try to equip pupils with the strategies they will find vital if they are going to be successful. The Skills lessons are only a part of this toolkit, but pupil feedback indicates they help dyslexic pupils as much if not more than others.

The final activity of the Skills course is to bring together, in a creative way, all the work done previously. The task is to work in groups to research and then produce a marketing document for what they consider to be "The best school in the world." You can imagine the nominations for Headteacher - I've only ever made it as caretaker!

I do not claim that all aspects of the course are particularly original and I have borrowed freely from many sources. Many teachers will be using the same techniques in their own classrooms or as part of PSE programmes and I have recently been accused of introducing The Literacy Hour into a secondary school! Whatever the case, I would like to think that the Skills lessons help all pupils, especially those with dyslexia, get closer to the target of "ability appropriate literacy."

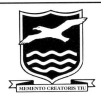

GRENVILLE COLLEGE
Bideford, Devon
EX39 3JR

CReSTeD Category B; Supporting Corporate Member of BDA

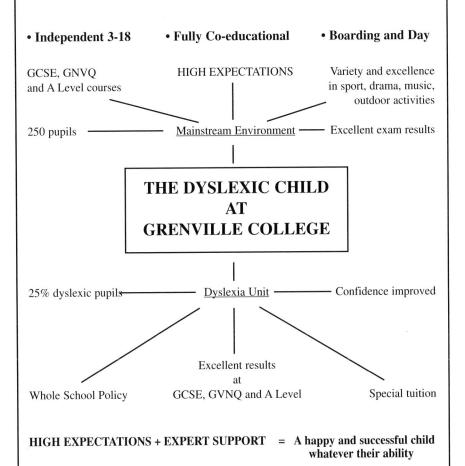

• **Independent 3-18**   • **Fully Co-educational**   • **Boarding and Day**

GCSE, GNVQ
and A Level courses

HIGH EXPECTATIONS

Variety and excellence
in sport, drama, music,
outdoor activities

250 pupils ———————— Mainstream Environment ——— Excellent exam results

THE DYSLEXIC CHILD
AT
GRENVILLE COLLEGE

25% dyslexic pupils————— Dyslexia Unit ————— Confidence improved

Excellent results
at
GCSE, GVNQ and A Level

Whole School Policy

Special tuition

HIGH EXPECTATIONS + EXPERT SUPPORT = **A happy and successful child
whatever their ability**

Telephone or fax for a prospectus, interview or a talk with the Head of the Dyslexia Unit
Tel: 01237 472212   *Fax: 01237 477020*
E-mail: info@grenville.devon.sch.uk   www: http://www.grenville.devon.sch.uk

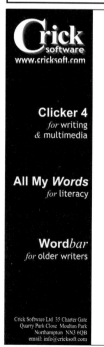
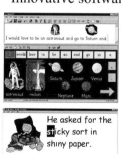

Hot tips for modern foreign languages (MFL)

Lyn Turnbull is the MFL tutor at Deeside College of Further Education, Deeside, Flintshire

You do not need to be super bright to learn a second (or third or fourth) language. It is perfectly possible and no big deal. So being dyslexic should not be a bar to becoming bi/multi-lingual. To argue that it is pointless to teach a child a MFL when he cannot cope with English is to miss the point about becoming the best you can be and allowing current problems in one area to inhibit progress in another. In fact the same argument could be used to justify disapplying a dyslexic child from Science or Geography!

Assume nothing

Although there will be many different starting points within a class, it is best to assume zero knowledge and begin with a level playing field for all. This approach allows natural abilities to shine through and perceived "learning difficulties" in other subjects may not become an issue in MFL learning.

Make it fun

Presenting MFL in the most positive light is a basic requirement. Ice breakers, games, activities borrowed from Drama etc will all go to put the target language in a meaningful context. Also this approach gives scope for oracy and minimises the need to write anything down. Indeed the less writing the better, especially in the early stages! "Information Gap" exercises, in which some class members have information needed by others, are particularly effective.

Mix up the learning styles

Looking for opportunities to include kinaesthetic, visual and auditory activities is a great boost to learning. This approach can also promote the very necessary repetition process while ringing the changes through learning styles.

KISS (keep it simple stupid)

Keep away from labels and jargon from as long as possible. Although, for example, masculine and feminine words are part of every European language except English, try to focus on the association of sounds ("la" with "Plage," "le" with "Poisson" rather than getting bogged down with genders. Multi-sensory approaches are powerful ways of making connections and encourage pupils to focus on differences. Often they will notice and comment upon gender differences long before the concept is formally introduced.

Opening up the ears

The ability to "hear" the sounds is fundamental to learning and this ability is not just the domain of non-dyslexics. Drawing pictures to link the sound to the word can be very useful as it allows learners to add their own interpretation. Playing with sounds is also helpful - in English, the word "people" may be presented as "pee - ople" - as is the use of mnemonics. Tapes are also invaluable.

Nurturing the delicate flowers

Dyslexic learners often bring a great deal of baggage to any sort of learning situation and nothing eases the load like success. Once MFL becomes associated with "I can" rather than "I can't" the sky can be the limit. Perhaps more than in any other subject it is important to set expectations and meaningful targets. Therefore warn pupils that "This bit is hard." but remind them of past successes with other hard bits and never miss the opportunity to point out that they will be better next lesson.

Being dyslexic has not prevented children from learning to speak their mother tongue efficiently, effectively and, in many cases, incessantly! It was learnt through saturation/repetition, love, persistence and because learning to say things achieved a result. By teaching the child, rather than the subject, there is no reason why dyslexic children cannot fulfil their potential in a modern foreign language and go on to make an impact in Europe and beyond. To deny them this opportunity would seem to be a high price to pay for a differently wired brain.

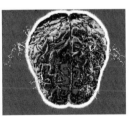

At school in two languages: dyslexia in Wales

When people talk about bilingual and multilingual teaching, and the difficulties that dyslexic (and other) children may meet when they have to learn in a second language, they are not usually thinking about Wales where the English and Welsh languages have equal status. At present some 20% of people speak Welsh as their first language and educational policies are vital to its preservation as a living, functional tongue. Here Ann Cooke takes a closer look.

Welsh and the National Curriculum

Welsh is a core subject in the National Curriculum in Wales and all children learn it to KS4. It may be taken as a first or as a learner's second language. For Welsh-speaking children in school where the teaching language is Welsh, English is introduced formally into the curriculum only after school year 2. Throughout Wales, Welsh is introduced as an oral language for English-speaking children from the early years. In some counties, especially in North and West Wales, it is also the medium of instruction for all children in the first years and this includes the introduction to reading and writing. The general objective is that all children should be bilingual orally, and on the way to use of the second language in its written form, by the time they are 11. They have therefore, two languages to master.

The use of Welsh varies throughout Wales, and the language pattern of schools reflects this. In some areas most children will be learning Welsh as a second language. In others, especially north-west and west Wales, the opposite may be more usual: Welsh first language children learning in Welsh;

others whose first language is English (though they may be Welsh by birth and so may their parents) possibly also learning in Welsh. Then there may be older children who have recently arrived in Wales, who are starting to learn Welsh at a later stage. Dyslexic children are to be found in all of these groups.

There is no simple comparison between the situation of children at school in Wales, and with starting a foreign language in Year 7. Wales is not a 'foreign' country. Welsh-speaking children hear English around them in the community and on the television. English first-language children are encouraged to attend Welsh playgroup and nursery school and they will begin oral Welsh in reception year.

Dyslexic children learning Welsh and English

Many dyslexic children learn to communicate in the second language without too much difficulty. More often than not, this all starts before there is any suspicion of a learning difficulty. Written Welsh has a very consistent spelling system, with a high level of phonic regularity. With few exceptions the sound-symbol correspondence is simple and unvarying. For that reason the language is easier to decode and write than English. It has been thought that children - regardless of home language - should find Welsh reading and writing easier for beginners to learn. It has also been thought that Welsh children learning in Welsh would not be 'dyslexic'. But these assume that dyslexia difficulties are due only to the difficulties of English. Welsh dyslexic children do struggle with reading in their first language. For instance, Welsh has far fewer short regular words. Even in reading books for young children the words can be varied and long. The grammatical constructions and mutations of Welsh (which cause words to change at the beginning and end) are difficult even for Welsh children.

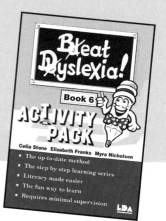

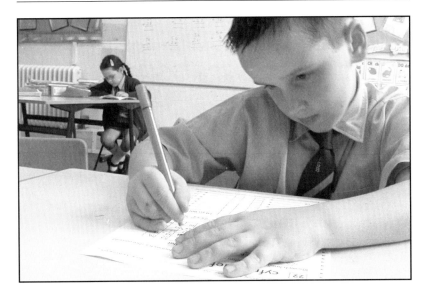

Both groups of children can have greater difficulties if they begin reading in their second language when their spoken vocabulary - and understanding - is limited and more problems can crop up when they begin reading in their first language. The writing systems of Welsh and English are different in many respects. Some consonants and many of the vowels are pronounced and spelled differently and this can be especially confusing for dyslexic children who do not easily master sound-to-letter correspondences.

Recognising the signs of dyslexia

All this has implications for the recognition of dyslexic children in Wales, especially at an early age. It is important to distinguish between a difficulty that comes from unfamiliarity with one of the languages and a difficulty in language learning itself. The level of language fluency is sometimes assumed to

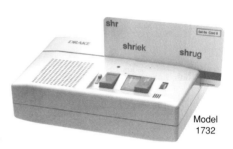

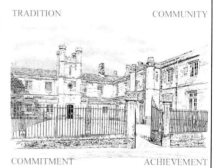

be the cause of the difficulty but waiting for the language to improve can result in damaging delay. It is important that teachers follow up early any signs that children may be meeting trouble. It is the same for Welsh children learning first in English: lack of progress has to be investigated and not put down to the difficulties of the language.

Assessment

There is a shortage of materials for assessment of children in Welsh. The British Ability Scales tests are often carried out using an informal translation, though there is no Welsh standardised version. Two screening tests, the Bangor Dyslexia Test (T.R. Miles) and the International Dyslexia Screening Test (Ian Smythe and Michael Davies) have recently been translated and are being tried out. There are standardised tests of reading, but only very recently has a spelling test been available (Prawf Glannau Menai- Gareth Payne, SEN Joint Committee, Gwynedd and Angelsey 1998). But as Welsh is such a regular language, children are often able to read at a level that puts them above the criteria for special needs help. It is important therefore that other aspects of language work are looked at carefully, particularly free writing where problems of grammar can be seen. Frequently dyslexic children get by in Welsh. It is when they run into problems with English that dyslexia is diagnosed, at which time it is realised that there are difficulties in their first language too.

Intervention

When help is set up for a dyslexic child, the language of the literacy programme has to be considered. Ideally, this will be the child's first language, so it can draw support from the oral language and vocabulary. But children in Wales who are Welsh

The Dyslexia Unit University of Wales Bangor

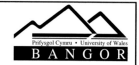

Prifysgol Cymru • University of Wales
B A N G O R

The Dyslexia Unit carries out a wide range of
work in the field of Dyslexia

Specialist teaching, including teaching in Welsh

(Unit teachers provide specialist services for Statemented dyslexic children
for three LEAs)

Support for dyslexic students at UWB

Consultation   Assessment

Specialist training courses (part-time) for teachers with QTS
(course members may qualify for BDA accreditations AMBDA and
ATS)

Research studies in collaboration with the School of Psychology

Director: Victor van Daal
Director of Teaching: Marie Jones
Director of Courses: Ann Cooke
Tutor/Counsellor for dyslexic students - Dorothy Gilroy
Consultation on Research - Professor Emeritus T.R. Miles
For information, phone Elizabeth Williams on 01248 382203
For training courses enquiries phone 01248 383841

The Dyslexia Unit is a Supporting Member of the BDA

learners may have particular needs. The language of instruction in their school may be Welsh and Welsh may be widely spoken in the local community. If they have already started reading in Welsh it may be better to continue until reading is established. When English is introduced the general phonic skills of blending and word-building should transfer to the new learning situation, even though the writing system is different and must now be learned.

Welsh language materials for children with special needs are not easy to find though they are increasing and there are some translations of English series (eg Skyways Books and Reading Tree). Specialist literacy materials - worksheets for reading and spelling work - are being produced including one (in press) by two teachers from the Bangor Dyslexia Unit. This is intended for use alongside the one structured phonic programme for Welsh children, O Gam i Gam, also by a Unit teacher. Materials are being produced by some county special needs teams, Swansea, Powys, Gwynedd and Mon SEN Advisory Service (Cumni Cynnal) among them. Whichever language is decided on, it is best to concentrate on one to start with, to avoid confusion.

It is also useful to look at how the child's education will go on in the longer term. If, for instance, he or she is going on to a Welsh-medium secondary school, competence in reading and writing in Welsh will be a high priority. Language matters should be considered when choosing schools, and whether parents will be able to help with homework. This could be especially important for a dyslexic child.

The addition of a third language when the child transfers to secondary school can place a heavy burden on the dyslexic pupil already coping with two languages. French is very demanding as it involves yet another phonic/phonetic system different from English and Welsh. German is a better option if it is offered.

None of this should affect the child's learning of spoken Welsh. Bilingualism is an enrichment and the dyslexic child should be encouraged to master the language orally. The children whose mother tongue is Welsh have an advantage here, as they will learn to speak English as a matter of course. For children from English first-language homes, becoming fully bilingual may be crucial if they want, eventually, to live and work in Wales.

Dyslexia Unit

University of Wales

Bangor

LL57 2DG

01248-383841/382203 (office)

Prosiect Dyslecsia Cymru

Amcan Prosiect Dyslecsia Cymru yw tynnu ynghyd y proffesiynolwyr sydd yn gweithio yn y maes dyslecsig, y sector fasnachol asiantaethau cyhoeddus, rhieni a gofalwyr, yn ychwanegol at unigolion dyslecsig i greu amgylchedd lle y gall yr unigolyn dyslecsig gyrraedd ei lawn botensial. Ceisir gwneud hyn drwy ddatblygu ymwybyddiaeth a dealltwriaeth, yn ychwanegol at ddarparu adnoddau i gefnogi'r unigolyn dyslecsig.

Am fanylion pellach, cysylltwch a:

Michael Davies

Rhif ffôn: 01239 682849

e-bost: llechryd@btinternet.com

The Welsh Dyslexia Project

The Welsh Dyslexia Project aims to bring together professionals working with the dyslexia community, the commercial sector, government agencies, parents and carer as well as dyslexic individuals to create an enviroment where the dyslexic individual may develop to their full potential. This will be facilitated through the development of awareness and understanding, as well as resources, for the support of the dyslexic individual.

For further details please contact Michael Davies

Tel:01239 682849

Email: llechryd@btinternet.com

How do I Google?

There are many search engines that one can use; the problem is deciding which is appropriate. Here, Ian Smythe looks at just one that he has found to be very useful.

For the first few years the Internet seemed to provide the perfect solution. Unfortunately, nobody had decided what the question was! Now we have lots of information, but it is a bit like a library that has no system, no order on the shelves. So how do you find anything. That is where the search engine comes in.

There are many search engines and meta search engines (these are search engines that look for your information by using many other search engines). One that provides an excellent service and is used by many professionals is Google. It can be found at

www.google.com

Why is it so good? Because it has very good search information and is incredibly quick. Part of the reason for that is that there are no adverts. It also has over 1,000,000,000 pages logged!

Improving your search

There are a number of tricks you can use to improve your search. Unfortunately they are different for every search engine. Here are the tips for Google. But most can be found in the section called "Advanced Searches".

A real example

In order to show how to use them, we shall take of teaching maths and dyslexia in the UK.

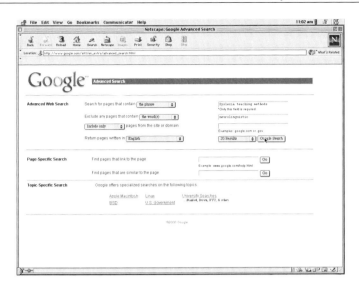

If you just typed in dyslexia, Google would offer 126,000 references. Other results are:

Dyslexia teaching (separate words) - 24,900

Dyslexia teaching (phrase) in English - 185

Dyslexia teaching (phrase) in English, excluding America - 169

In the search box you will find the terms

"dyslexia teaching" -America

Now type in the following "+maths" to give

"dyslexia teaching" -America +maths

This reduces it down to just 15 results, a very manageable number!

One more trick - click on the words "similar pages" that are after each link.

(Please note that this does not suggest an endorsement of the results, nor necessarily the best source for this subject! See this Handbook for ideas.)

Reading Difficulties – Listening Books can help

Listening Books has provided a postal talking book library service for almost fifty years. This type of resource can open up the magic world of reading to those with specific learning difficulties, including dyslexia, for whom reading print is frustrating, even impossible.

Listening Books has three digital recording studios and record books in their entirety, eg, classics, history, poetry, biographies, autobiographies, science, travel, and dramatizations in addition to well-known novels, sci-fi, general fiction and other pleasurable reading.

The Young Peoples' Library makes sure that young dyslexic individuals can enjoy the very best of both classic and contemporary reading. That way they have access to the stories that lie at the heart of a literate future. Listening to books can be a great way to focus and develop your imagination and creative skills.

Listening Books is an easy to operate talking books library. Members receive a catalogue from which they can make their selection on the enclosed order form.

Cassettes are sent out promptly (by Freepost) and the library staff are always on hand to answer questions. Membership of Listening Books costs £50 per annum (less than £1 per week) for individual members and £100 per annum for corporate membership.

For further information contact the Membership Department at Listening Books on 020 7407 9417 or writing to Listening Books, 12 Lant Street, London SE1 1QH or on their website www.listening-books.org.uk

Disabled Students Allowance (DSA)

Jane Myers give a brief overview of the DSA.

Students in Higher Education, who have been formally assessed as dyslexic, can apply to their Local Education Authority for a Disabled Students Allowance. From September 2000, part-time students, studying at least 50% of a full-time course leading to a degree, and post graduate students, will be eligible for this allowance. This can cover any supportive materials, particularly ICT for dyslexics.

For more information about the DSA, students should contact the Disability Officer within their college or university. The Officer responsible for dyslexia should be contacted as soon as possible after a place has been accepted.

The LEA will need evidence of dyslexia from a qualified psychologist experienced in working with dyslexic adults or a report from someone with a qualification from a professional training course involving the assessment of adults with dyslexia, such as the OCR (formerly RSA) Diploma in Specific Learning Difficulties, may be accepted. The LEA will usually expect evidence of an assessment done in the last two years. The report should say why special equipment or support is considered necessary. An ACCESS Centre can offer a full assessment of a student's needs and requirements, including ICT needs. The DSA is no longer means tested.

Value of the DSA for the academic year 2000/2001

- equipment allowance can be up to £4,155. It is a once only payment.

- general allowance can be up to £1,385 per year. This is to cover such things as tape cassettes, electronic spellchecker, calculator or the cost of photocopying etc.

- non-medical helper's allowance can be up to £10,505 per year. This could cover salary costs for a reader who records text for the student to hear, or for a note taker, typist or a support teacher.

Questions which might be asked

The LEA will consider certain points when determining suitability for DSA:

- What course are you doing?

- What facilities does the college or university have to offer you?

- What are the ICT requirements for your course and university?

- What is the suitability of ICT to be supplied?

- Are you IT literate?

Here are some questions which may wish to ask to ensure you receive the right equipment.

- Is there enough memory?

- Will there be a scanner and printer?

- Who will offer me support if anything goes wrong with the ICT?

- Can I have training so that I get the most out of my ICT?

- Will I be supplied with paper, ink cartridges, disks etc?

Try and buy your equipment from one dealer. Ask the dealer to show you the software working. This will help ensure that software is compatible. Ask for the correct warranties, this will help you if anything goes wrong.

For further information on student allowances contact:

The DfEE Tel: 0800 731 9133. (for students only)

Leaflet 'Bridging The Gap - A Guide To Disabled Students Allowance (DSAs) in higher education in 2000/2001'.

Web: http://www.dfee.gov.uk/support/support2000/ch05.htm

Other Useful contacts

SKILL - The National Bureau for Students with Disabilities

Skill has helpful general information and literature, especially about allowances for disabled students.

Tel: 0800 328 5050

Fax: 020 7450 0650

E-mail: info@skill.org.uk

Web: http://www.skill.org.uk/

The Educational Grants Advisory Service (EGAS) offers funding guidance about loans, grants and benefits from educational trusts and charities for disadvantaged students over 16.

Send an SAE to 501-505 Kingsland Road, London, E8 4AU for a form for completion, to enable EGAS to give you appropriate advice.

Tel: 020 7249 6636   Fax: 020 7249 5443

Dyslexic Pupils and Statutory Assessment: Key Stages 1, 2 and 3

Dyslexic children can, and do, perform well in national tests. Test situations are not easy for children with specific learning difficulties. However, it is important to know that the special arrangements give them a chance to compete on equal terms to that of their peers. Mel Lever looks at what can be done.

SATs

The facts given below are taken from material provided for schools by the Qualifications and Curriculum Authority (ref: QCA/99/428, QCA/99/429, QCA/98/246). Some instructions have been paraphrased; others are quoted verbatim.

Permission for special arrangements

In 2000 permission for special arrangements for children taking KS 2 and 3 tests had to be requested, in writing, by 11th February, schools being notified of decisions by 14th April (KS2) or 7th April (KS3).

The QCA documents, entitled Assessment and Reporting Arrangements for the Key Stages 1, 2 and 3 Tests in 2000, give clear directions:

"The tasks and tests are intended to assess children's ability in a fair and comparable way and so that as many children as possible have access to them. They are designed so that many children with special educational needs can undertake them in their standard format...... teachers may need to adapt the administrative arrangements for the tasks and tests so that some children can demonstrate their achievement.....

adaptations should neither advantage nor disadvantage individual children." (Key Stage 1)

"The tests are designed to be accessible to the vast majority of children.... When considering making special arrangements, the focus should be on the assessment needs of the individual child. Special consideration cannot be applied retrospectively during the marking process.... Special arrangements must not provide an unfair advantage. It is, therefore, important to ensure that any support given does not alter the nature of the test questions, and that all answers given are the child's own." (Key Stages 2 and 3)

The documents list categories of pupils for whom special arrangements can be made:

- children with a statement of special education needs, or who are shown on the school's special needs register at stage 4 of the SEN Code of Practice;

- children who are shown on the school's special needs register at stage 3 or below of the SEN Code of Practice, and whose learning difficulty or disability significantly affects access to the tests;

- children who are unable to sit and work at a test for a sustained period because of a disability or emotional, social or behavioural difficulties;

- children for whom English is an additional language and who have limited fluency in English.

Dyslexic pupils qualify under the first two categories. Many would qualify under the others too.

Children may be disapplied temporarily or permanently from taking the tests (or tasks). "This may be done in one of two ways:

- through section 364 of the Education Act 1996, which

specifies that some or all of the national curriculum may be modified or disapplied by a child's statement of special educational needs; or

• through section 365 of the Education Act 1996, which specifies that some or all of the national curriculum may be temporarily disapplied for a child."

There are set procedures that the headteacher must follow to disapply children. These include discussion with the parents. Upon deciding to disapply a child the head must write a special direction; one copy goes in the child's educational records, one to at least one of the child's parents, one to the chair of the governing body and one to the LEA. Parents have a right of appeal against any decision. In such a case they should ask the school to explain the procedure for parental requests and appeals as outlined in the documents.

What special arrangements may be made?

Allowing additional time during the tests

"Up to 25 per cent additional time may be given for the written tests at the school's discretion for a child with a statement or at stage 4 of the SEN Code of Practice. Requests for additional time must be made for all other children. Additional time will be allowed, for example, where a child has a physical or sensory difficulty or has a specific learning difficulty which significantly affects the speed of his or her reading or writing…. For children who are likely to experience fatigue, it may be appropriate to separate the tests into sections, either instead of, or as well as, providing additional time."

"For the mental arithmetic test, children at any stage of the SEN Code of Practice who do not have visual impairment, hearing impairment or motor disabilities are not allowed any

SIBFORD SCHOOL

Sibford Ferris, Banbury, Oxon OX15 5QL
Tel: 01295 781200 - Fax: 01295 781204
Email: Sibford.School@dial.pipex.com   www.sibford.oxon.sch.uk
Co-Educational Day and Boarding School with a unique Quaker ethos
Founded in 1842   SHMIS   320 pupils 5-18

- A dyslexia friendly school - CReSTeD Category B
- Small class sizes - Teacher to pupil ratio of 1 : 8
- Specialist Dyslexia teaching includes Maths and Speech & Language provision
- Information Technology across the curriculum
- Sixth Form courses leading to A level and GNVQ
- Excellence in Arts, Music, Drama and Technology

At Sibford School the dyslexic child gains confidence and self-esteem, supported by the school's ethos of treating each child as an individual.

~ each TALENTED ~ each DIFFERENT ~ all VALUED ~

contact the Admissions Secretary for details at
SIBFORD SCHOOL
Registered Charity No. 1068256

SLINDON COLLEGE

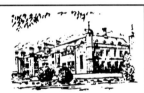

Slindon, Arundel, West Sussex
CReSTeD Category C accredited

A boarding and day school for boys aged 9 - 16
- A beautiful environment in which to learn and develop
- Small classes (10-12 pupils) and individual attention
- EXPERT help from our LEARNING SUPPORT DEPARTMENT for Dyslexia and ADD/ADHD.
- Full or flexi-boarding and day places.
- An excellent broad based curriculum, including rural studies, automotive engineering, home economics, photography and PE.
- Masses of extra-curricular activities including Combined Cadet Force, D of E Award scheme, motor vehicle maintenance, a variety of sport & involvement in our animal kingdom.
- Strong pastroal support within a caring family environment.

For further details, an informal chat, or to arrange a visit please telephone Jenny Davies, Registrar on 01243 814320, or
email: registrar@slindoncollege.fsnet.co.uk

additional time as a few additional seconds are unlikely to be helpful." (KS2, KS3)

Dyslexic children may need more time to read papers, may be slow at working out and writing down answers. They may need adult help with reading and writing (see below). At Fairley House we have found it useful to have the extra time available, although not all children take advantage of it. Some children use the time well in all papers, some need extra time in one or two papers only. If a child has a reading difficulty then extra time in the English papers will not always be of use. The intensity of test taking also means that some dyslexic children are unable to carry on for much longer than the intended time, even when papers are split into sections.

Specific arrangements

"Care has been taken to ensure the language used in the papers is as straightforward as possible and that the questions allow access to the test materials for the maximum number of children. Therefore, school-based adaptations to the test papers must not involve re-wording of questions but may include the following arrangements." (KS2, KS3)

Separating the tests into sections

"No permission is required for this specific arrangement. Schools do not need to apply for permission to separate the tests into sections, but must ... The overall time given to a child for the test should remain the same as if the test had not been separated into sections. It is important that children have the opportunity to attempt all parts of a paper so that the test properly reflects their attainment. If children are given rest breaks, this time must not be used to discuss the contents of the test." (KS2, KS3)

Parents of dyslexic children in the mainstream school, who feel that this arrangement would be useful to their child, should discuss it at an early date with the child's headteacher.

Making taped versions for the written tests

"No permission is required for this specific arrangement. Schools may provide taped versions of the written mathematics and science tests where a child would normally be given such support, or have access to the regular provision of readers as part of normal classroom practice. The taped versions must be provided in the medium of English. Taped versions of the English tests are not allowed.

"For mathematics and science, the general instructions may be clarified on the taped versions, but no other modification to the wording must take place. Taped versions can also be used in conjunction with modified versions of the tests. When taped versions have been prepared, children should be given opportunities to become familiar with using tapes before the tests so that they can show their best work in the time available. Practice tapes used for this purpose must not be based on the content of any of the current year's tests."

(KS2, KS3)

Taped versions can be very useful for dyslexic children. Teachers and parents need to discuss whether it would be more appropriate for a child to have a taped version or to have extra help through a reader. The choice depends very much on what happens in the normal class life of the child and how the child reacts to specific help.

Photocopying onto coloured paper or using coloured overlays

"No permission is required for this specific arrangement.... Coloured overlays and coloured filter lenses may also be used." (KS2, KS3)

Some dyslexic children are helped by coloured overlays or filter lenses. Where these are used as part of the normal day, they should be used in the tests.

Presentation of diagrams

"No permission is required for this specific arrangement. The shading on diagrams, including charts and graphs, may be enhanced to increase visual clarity. Bold lines may also be added for children with spatial perception difficulties..... Diagrams may be enlarged, cut out, embossed or mounted on card or other material, according to usual practice in the classroom. However, considerable care should be taken in order to avoid altering the nature of any question, particularly in mathematics. Diagrams must not be altered in any other way." (KS2, KS3)

Use of apparatus, materials and other aids

"No permission is required for this specific arrangement. In mathematics and science, teachers may wish to provide real objects which look like those illustrated in the tests. In mathematics, care must be taken to use shapes identical to those drawn and to keep relative sizes the same. It is not expected that children will have number apparatus in the tests. However, in individual cases, for those few children who may initially need support, structured number apparatus such as Dienes blocks may be provided if this is normal classroom practice. Counters should not be used as they do not provide appropriate support." (KS2, KS3)

"For questions involving symmetry, pupils may be given

mirrors and tracings of the shapes in the question papers." (KS3)

"In science, the apparatus or materials illustrated in the question paper may be shown to children. Children must not, however, experiment with the apparatus." (KS2, KS3)

"Mechanical and technological aids normally used by children, including word processors, may be used for all tests except the English handwriting test. However, in English, spellcheckers must not be used in the spelling and the level 6 extension tests." (KS2) Such aids are also available for KS3 tests. No spellcheckers can be used and "the assessment of pupils' writing will be based on aspects of the performance criteria other than handwriting."

Use of dictionaries and spellcheckers

"Dictionaries, word lists and thesauri are not allowed in the English reading test, spelling test or the English extension test. Dictionaries may be used in the writing test, if this is normal classroom practice, however, thesauri may not be used in the writing test. Spellcheckers may be used in any test except the spelling test and level 6 English extension test.

"Given the nature of the mental arithmetic test, word lists are inappropriate and may not be used.

"Monolingual dictionaries and thesauri are not allowed in the mathematics and science tests as they could provide an unfair advantage to children.

"Spellcheckers may be used in any of the mathematics and science tests." (KS2)

Use of readers

"Schools do not need to apply for permission to use a reader in the mathematics and science tests, unless this leads to a request for additional time. Readers may be used in the mathematics and science tests but must not be used in the English tests, except for help with reading general instructions.

"Readers should normally be teachers or support assistants, but need not be teachers of the subject being tested... Readers should be familiar with the format and style of the tests, and be briefed about their own role and about any subject-specific issues which might arise during the tests.... Permission for early opening will not be granted for the preparation of readers." (KS2, KS3)

At Fairley House we have found that the use of readers is necessary for, and acceptable to, the children. Our children are used to having such help and do not shirk putting their hands up to ask! Where children are known to need help with all reading they are allocated a specific helper. Many children need help with particular words. This means that we have several teachers and assistants on hand to help.

Use of amanuenses

"Schools do not need to apply for permission to use an amanuensis in the English, mathematics and science tests, unless this leads to a request for additional time. An amanuensis may be used for any of the tests except for the handwriting test. However, in the writing test and the English level 6 extension test [in KS2], an amanuensis may be used only for a child who is unable to write down his or her own answers or use a word processor. If a child is unable to take the handwriting test, the external marker will award an average mark for handwriting. If an amanuensis is used for the spelling test, the child should be asked to spell out each word to the amanuensis. This may mean he or she needs to be tested in a separate room. Where an amanuensis has been used in the mathematics tests, the same support should be used for the science tests. The amanuensis should ensure that all language, punctuation and phrasing are the child's own. Particular care should be taken when following a child's instructions to draw on diagrams, charts and graphs in mathematics and science.

"External marking agencies will supply a form for schools to use for this purpose. If an amanuensis has been used, the form supplied by the external marking agency for this purpose should be attached to the child's test papers when these are sent to the external marker." (KS2, similar wording in KS3)

Transcripts

"No permission is required for this specific arrangement. A transcript should be made only when it would be very difficult for the external marker to read a child's handwriting. The child's original paper must always be sent to the marker with the transcript. The transcript should be made as soon as possible after the child has completed a test. The child should be asked to read his or her work to the adult making the transcript, but care must be taken to ensure that no original answers are altered at this stage. A transcript may show spelling corrected from the child's original script, provided the child has read out the correct word to the adult who is transcribing his or her answers. All punctuation and phrasing must be the child's own." (KS2, KS3)

At Fairley House we have found that most children like to write as much as possible on their own. We transcribe words that we feel an external examiner would not be able to read, or write some whole sentences in the science and mathematics papers where appropriate. Because of their touchtyping skills, children do not normally ask for help with the written English papers.

Taking the tests in a separate room or away from school

"No permission is required for this specific arrangement. The use of a separate room may allow the school to meet the needs of a child who finds it hard to concentrate for long periods and who requires rest breaks or additional time." (KS2, KS3)

Special arrangements for the mental arithmetic test

The taped version of the mental arithmetic test must be administered to all children unless they require specific support [e.g. visually impaired or hearing impaired pupils, or those with a motor disability]. It is anticipated that such children will be either at stage 4 or above of the SEN Code of Practice or will be children for whom English is an additional language. Headteachers must ensure that the special arrangements outlined in this section are used only in appropriate cases. The test must be administered on a specific day in early May (please check with QCA for dates). In cases where the test is required to be administered individually or in small groups, the headteacher must ensure that children do not have the opportunity to discuss the contents of the mental arithmetic test until it has been administered to all children.

"With the exception of children identified in this section, no additional time may be granted for the mental arithmetic test. Children on the SEN Code of Practice at stage 4 or above, or those granted additional time in the main written tests, are not automatically entitled to additional time in the mental arithmetic test." (KS2, KS3)

GCSE and GCE

The information below is taken from material provided for schools by the Joint Forum for General Qualifications: Examinations and Assessment for GCSE and GCE:

Regulations and Guidance relating to Candidates with Special Requirements 2000.

Permission for special arrangements

"The awarding bodies recognise that there are some candidates who have coped with the learning demands of a course but for whom the standard arrangements for the assessment of their attainment may present a barrier.... It is the responsibility of the Head of Centre (e.g. Headteacher, Principal) entering a candidate to ensure that any request on behalf of a candidate is based on firm evidence of an unfair barrier to assessment of attainment." (p 2)

Special arrangements may be made for pupils with specific learning difficulties. The document lists difficulties included reading accuracy, reading speed, spelling, handwriting speed, handwriting legibility, attention and concentration, clumsiness and disorganisation. The Head must support requests for special arrangements, the Examining Bodies being responsible for the consideration and approval of such requests. Specific enquiries should be addressed to the particular Examining Body conducting the examinations, general enquiries to the Joint Forum. A need for special arrangements must be related to specific examination papers and/or other forms of assessment. Dyslexic pupils may not need special arrangements in all subjects.

A Statement does not automatically qualify a candidate for special arrangements; possible needs should be considered at the annual Review before coursework commences. The decision regarding special arrangements will rest with the Examining Body, who will take into consideration the candidate's usual method of working in the classroom. Any request for special arrangements for candidates with specific learning difficulties must be supported by evidence derived from an educational psychologist or an appropriately qualified teacher. A Psychological Assessment Report form is available in the document. The Examining Body will need historical evidence of the candidate's needs and an indication of how these are met; arrangements requested for the examination must reflect past and present needs.

What special arrangements may be made?

Additional time, up to 25% of the total examination time, may be allowed in most subjects, but not normally in a component where performance of a task in a limited time is an assessment objective. This may be granted by the Head of Centre without application to the awarding body. In exceptional cases more than 25% additional time may be allowed. However, the document points out that too much time may be counter-productive. Supervised breaks or rest periods may be given; such time will not be deducted from the extra time allowed.

Questions may be read to candidates except where understanding of the written word is being assessed. Standardised reading tests should be used to demonstrate a candidate's difficulties. Any request would need to provide psychological evidence of a discrepancy between reading ability and reasoning ability, and a Reading Age of 12.0 years and below for GCE and 10.0 years and below for GCSE.

A typewriter, word processor or other aid may be used by candidates who are unable to write, or who need such support during the examinations. (Printing of answers may take place after the time allowed has expired.) Spell-checks, thesauri or similar electronic devices may not normally be used. A word processor is not allowed where a significant proportion of marks are allocated to handwriting and presentation skills. In such a case a verbatim transcript is allowed; samples of work may be required by the Examining Board. Dictionaries and spell-checks may be used in coursework unless a set task specifically excludes their use. Coursework produced on a computer may be required to be submitted for inspection by a Moderator.

If a candidate is exempted from the assessment of spelling, punctuation and grammar, and compensation given in the form of an adjustment to marks, an indication to this effect will be made on the certificate. However, no exemption from this assessment will be allowed in English. Pupils may be exempted from such assessment in English Literature, resulting in an indication on the certificate.

An amanuensis may be used if responses cannot be communicated through other means. In this case, candidates will not be expected to dictate spelling and punctuation. Examples of the candidate's written work under controlled conditions may be offered as evidence. Because literacy skills are being assessed, candidates with specific learning difficulties taking English will not be allowed the use of an amanuensis. In English Literature, such use may be permitted in exceptional cases.

Conclusion

National tests are a valuable way of assessing the ability of children compared with their peers. Teachers and parents of dyslexic children need to be aware of the many ways that they can be helped to take part in the tests taking advantage of the special arrangements as set out in the documents. It is important to note the dates when special arrangements can be requested and granted. Special needs cannot be discussed after the tests have been taken.

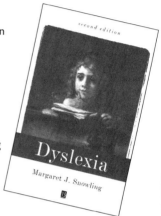

Creating a dyslexia friendly school

When Elizabeth Henderson talks about making a school dyslexia friendly, she is in fact talking about how she makes it friendly for all pupils. Here she shares some of her thoughts on how to achieve this.

Let's pretend for a moment that I am a doctor and not the headteacher of a primary school.

> *There is a condition that has been the subject of research for over a hundred years. It affects about 20% of all people, adult and children alike, to one degree or another. It has been of interest to a wide range of academic disciplines, many of which have produced findings that can be directly related to different, but successful, forms of treatment and therapy. There now exists well-researched, accessible and effective ways of helping those who have the condition. These treatments are not very expensive or difficult to provide. Clearly I have a professional responsibility to know about this condition, about how to identify it in my patients, to provide appropriate courses of therapy and treatment, to monitor the success of these actions and to ensure that other professionals in my practice do the same.*

But I am headteacher of an ordinary primary school. The condition I am referring to is dyslexia. My professional responsibilities remain the same as they are in my imagined scenario above. That is why I feel so passionately that teachers and headteachers are doing the right thing when they work together to create schools that are 'dyslexia friendly'.

As with the management of ALL change in a school, the headteacher is most successful when he/she has a clear vision which stays in place. My objective has been that I want to create schools that make good provision for ALL children, including those that are dyslexic. These children form the bulk of all schools' Special Needs registers.

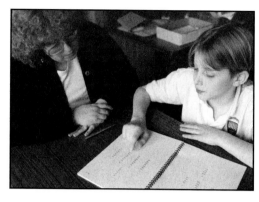

(Remember that figure of 20%: Martin Turner and Margaret Newton's research have both produced the same figure. The smaller 10% often quoted, refers to only the more seriously dyslexic students.) The teaching approaches that suit them best are also excellently effective for all other pupils in the school.

Before setting about the task in hand it may be helpful to see the model that I believe has helped my pupils and the staff in my schools. To bring in some realism and practical help I will also discuss some of the difficulties that have occurred and how they have been overcome.

Issue

Many schools have 'pockets' of knowledge about dyslexia and how best to teach those with dyslexic ways of learning. Children can do well or badly according to the teacher they have for the year.

Action

Whole-school philosophy and policy written with staff and governors, including high expectations for the rate of change, opportunities for the 'vision' to be constantly redefined, a requirement that the headteacher is seen to be helping and watching in a cooperative and professional way every day.

Problem

Some staff who may be resistant to change in general or this philosophy in particular will need a combination of enthusiastic encouragement, good practical support and, if necessary, a requirement, that their teaching takes account of the change in the school's focus onto dyslexic pupils.

Outcome

Everyone in the school has a good understanding of the nature of dyslexia, that they cooperate successfully together to enable all the dyslexic children to feel and become effective learners and balanced people.

Issue

Generally speaking teachers have not been trained to teach dyslexic children. They can feel threatened by the levels of knowledge amongst parents and other professionals. Teachers' Assistants are often key workers with these children and frequently say they feel badly equipped to help.

Action

One or two whole school training days (to include all Teachers' Assistants and volunteers) can be the most cost effective way of overcoming the problem. Courses can be 'bought-in' from specialist training centres (Helen Arkell, Hornsby, Dyslexia Institute and many others.) It is also good to offer as many teachers as possible, additional and more specialist courses to enable them to return to school with higher levels of knowledge and skill to pass on to their colleagues.

Problem

Funding for these courses may be a problem, but I have found our local Further Education College courses relatively affordable and very good. Pockets of DfEE and Standards funding can be well used for this purpose.

Outcome

Entire staff very knowledgeable and skillful in using multisensory and other dyslexia friendly techniques and approaches. A shared interest and enthusiasm that grows from increased practical knowledge that can be seen to benefit the children.

Issue

However skilled, efficient and hardworking the teacher, ONE teacher cannot provide appropriate amounts of time or help to cater for the learning needs of the wide range of abilities in a class. The combination of the new Curriculum 2000 and the requirement to provide for a much wider range of special educational needs makes it impossible to teach classes of over fifteen children without the help of another adult who is trained and adept at supporting the teacher, every morning.

Action

Plan the budget for the year ahead to enable the school to employ this level of assistance for the teachers. Ensure the school provides appropriate training, access to structured support materials and ongoing frequent meetings to address worries and concerns.

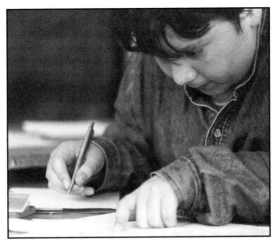

Problem

Governors particularly, can be unaware of the enormous value good Teachers' Assistants can offer the school. The reasons behind the headteacher's desire to increase the levels of classroom support can be seen clearly if Governors visit the school during the morning sessions, when National Literacy Strategy and National Numeracy Strategy are in progress. Whatever other demands there are on the budget, little else will improve the quality of education for so many children than this one measure.

Outcome

All classes will be able to provide appropriately differentiated levels of work in numeracy and literacy. There will be a skilled adult to help all groups more often and children will have access to assistance when they begin to worry about their work or when they need extra help. Standards will improve and staff morale with them.

Issue

Parents of children with learning difficulties often feel unsupported by their school. They do not know how to help their child, or the exact nature of his/her difficulties.

Action

If the whole-school philosophy is shared with parents and termly discussion groups are organised for them to air their worries and share their solutions with each other, they know that the school is 'on their side'. Contact becomes informal, relaxed and helpful to all concerned. Paperwork is kept to a satisfactory working minimum so that it informs when necessary, but does not distract staff from the teaching and caring role that is so much more important.

Problem

Good quality contact with parents is time consuming and all staff can benefit from Time-Management training to ensure they make appropriate time available to parents without endangering their private and professional time allocations.

Outcome

Parents will work with the school and its staff. They will be relaxed and well informed about the nature of their child's difficulties. They will be expected and willing to help in practical ways to improve the standards of learning in their child.

Issue

Dyslexic children often show signs of low self-esteem by behaving badly, becoming the class clown, repeatedly getting into tiffs and arguments in the playground, bullying or becoming the object of bullying or becoming very withdrawn and shy. Their progress at school and the fact that they feel as if they must be 'thick', contribute to their feelings of failure and add to the chances of them becoming under confident in the way they behave.

Action

The school can provide an environment where dyslexic children feel as valued as others if everyone has opportunities to be able to be good at whatever they find easy. Weekly chances for all the pupils to talk about their out-of-school activities and to perform skills or display their knowledge to others will ensure that they and their peers appreciate that each of us is different and that we ALL have our own set of aptitudes and abilities. The academic children are often praised in the lessons in the school environment, but subjects like Design and Technology, Music, Art, Drama, Games and P.E. are where the dyslexic children often 'shine'. Appropriate value and appreciation of their skills will enhance their self-esteem, but it will also encourage all pupils to value each other's abilities.

Problem

The national emphasis at present is very strongly on test results in the Core subjects. It is easy for teachers and parents to lose sight of the 'whole child' in their efforts to help the child to gain higher marks in these subjects. League tables may enable the government of the day to demonstrate that their policies are improving education, but well educated and balanced citizens are what the country needs.

Outcome

The school builds a reputation for having confident, bright, happy and contributing pupils, whatever their own skills and abilities. The dyslexic ones know that they have a

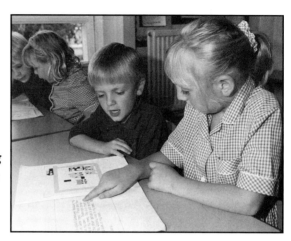

different learning style, but learn to work around it successfully. They, and all the other pupils respect each other for their individual differences.

Dyslexia friendly schools are active and interesting places in which to work, in my experience, because everyone in the institution, adults and children alike, feel valued, committed, challenged and respected as individuals. Dyslexia is no longer seen as an abnormality or difference, it is just one of the normal attributes one finds in people in the real world.

Cameron House

4 The Vale, London SW3 6AH.
Tel: 020 7352 4040
Fax: 020 7352 2349
E-mail: cameronhouse@lineone.net

Principal: Mrs J. M. Ashcroft, BSc, Dip.Ed., Member of IAPS
Headmistress: Miss F.N. Stack BA PGCE, Member of IAPS
Type: London Day School, Co-Educational, 4 - 11 years
Entry at 4 and at any stage from 4 upwards
No of Pupils: 110

Fees per Term: £2180-£2300

Religious Affiliation: Church of England - all religions welcome

• Small Classes taught by highly qualified, experienced staff. Specialists teach French, Music, Sport, Swimming, Art and Pottery.

• An exciting variety of after school clubs, e.g. Art, Karate, Fencing, Football, Chess, Ballet, Music and French.

• Field Trips and excursions part of the school curriculum.

• Children prepared for external examinations to London day and boarding schools.

• Provision for bright dyslexics

For details call the School Secretary on 020 7352 4040

DYSLEXIA:
At the dawn of the new century
18–21 April 2001

Dyslexia at work:
do I tell or don't I tell?

It can be very intimidating to approach an employer and divulge sensitive information about yourself. There are many reasons for not telling people about your dyslexia. It is a very personal matter. Jane Myers looks at what to consider when asking yourself this question.

This article cannot tell you whether you should or should not tell; ultimately this is your decision. Generally you will know when the time is right or whether the situation is safe for you to volunteer this information. As we know, dyslexic people can often be very intuitive. So use your intuition to assess how people might react to this news. Consider carefully how they might respond to the issues surrounding dyslexia.

For some people, explaining about dyslexia can be relatively easy. However, revealing information about your strengths and weaknesses can leave you feeling vulnerable and open to discrimination. It is difficult to predict other people's reactions to your dyslexia, particularly if they do not know much about it.

For many adults, their dyslexia will not have been recognised in school. Prior to discussing your dyslexia with a line manager it may be worth considering whether a diagnosis would be useful. A specialist teacher assessment or an Educational Psychologist's assessment would provide you with a report which would then help you explain your dyslexia to your employer. You do not need to share the whole document with the employer, but sections or notes from such a paper may be useful in discussions. To be covered by the DDA, you would require an assessment or some evidence of your difficulty.

If you discover your dyslexia whilst in a current job, your employer may support you through an assessment, possibly allowing time away from work or actually paying for the assessment.

Remember, this is a difficult decision and it is yours alone. Some adult dyslexics choose not to inform their employers about their dyslexia; it is not compulsory.

Considerations

It may be worth considering the following points...

- Does the employer have a good track record of supporting people with disabilities?

- How much does the employer know about dyslexia?

- Can adjustments really be made? Can they be made with ease?

- Will the adjustments really make a difference?

- What are your difficulties? Are they really a difficulty within your job?

- Is your dyslexia really causing you a problem within the workplace?

What are the benefits of telling your employer about your dyslexia?

When an employer has some knowledge of dyslexia and is pro-active about supporting staff, there may be:

- greater understanding

- improved communication

- equal opportunities

- Appropriate career enhancement.

- Adjustments to accommodate needs.

- Increased understanding and appreciation of abilities.

- Improved work environment.

- Appreciation of how different stresses may affect your work.

- Support.

- Access to grants for support , i.e. software, secretarial help.

- Cover against discrimination by the Disability Discrimination Act 1995.

- Confidence.

What does the employer gain by knowing about your dyslexia?

- Better communication.

- Improved work environment.

- Improved productivity.

- Getting the most out of their workforce.

- Understanding the different qualities that employees have to offer.

- Greater understanding of the workforce.

- Development of trust and honesty.

- Flexibility all round.

- An appreciation of the employee's openness and honesty.

What can go wrong?

A major concern expressed by a number of adults is that they will be labelled - only ever being seen as a dyslexic and not as an individual.

This is suggesting a rather negative view of the situation but it does recognise potential areas of difficulty which are worth considering.

• Misunderstanding

• Discrimination

• Lack of communication

• Loss of confidence

• Bullying

• Intimidation

• Unsuitable career enhancement – if any

Be positive:-

• Educate your employer about dyslexia.

• Provide employers with information about yourself.

• Explain how dyslexia affects you personally.

• Sell your dyslexia as an asset to your employer.

• Sell your strengths

• Highlight what you can do; do not list what you find difficult.

• Whenever you mention a weakness, explain how you compensate for it.

• Discuss how your workplace could be improved to accommodate your needs.

- Be open about your dyslexia.
- Find out about grants and funds that can be adapted to your needs.
- Be prepared for lots of questions; encourage discussion.
- Be positive!

Appreciate that this is a two way deal; if your employer is prepared to make adjustments for you, be prepared to work a little harder or to fit into a new system. If an employer is prepared to buy new software, make the effort to use it to its full capacity.

Here are some facts which might help your decision...

- Dyslexia is covered by the Disability Discrimination Act 1995 (DDA).
- The DDA prohibits discrimination against disabled people in employment
- An employer has a duty to make reasonable adjustments if a disabled employee is at a substantial disadvantage in relation to a non-disabled person.
- An employer must not refuse to employ someone simply because they have a disability. They also have a duty to think about different ways of working.

Note 1 - The Act does not apply to the police, armed services personnel, prison officers, fire fighters or people who work on board ships, aircraft or hovercraft. It does not apply to organisations that have fewer than 15 employees.

However, it would be fair to say that some of these employers do make conscious efforts to accommodate a dyslexic person within the workplace. The Army is an excellent example of creating a service wide policy and strategy to offer support to dyslexic personnel.

Note 2 - if you do not declare your dyslexia and subsequently feel discriminated against, it would be more difficult to prove a case under the DDA. The employer should be given the opportunity to make adjustments to accommodate the dyslexic employee before taking a case against them for discrimination.

Employers must not discriminate against a disabled person in the:

• recruitment and retention of employees

• promotion and transfers

• training and development

• the dismissal process

It is worth stressing to an employer that adjustments required for dyslexic people are not usually expensive. A willingness to be flexible is the most important thing. Dyslexic people will want their employer to understand their dyslexia so they can feel confident about discussing any difficulties that arise. They may ask an employer to be flexible about some paperwork or provide suitable ICT.

Remember –

It's your choice to tell,

It may well be to your advantage,

Your career may progress more positively,

You are covered by the DDA95 if you do tell,

You may lose out if you do not tell,

Telling is not compulsory.

Your career

If you are having difficulty at work, are you sure you are in the right job?

Often people dive into a career because it sounds ideal for them and it's what they have always wanted to do. However, many jobs contain hidden paperwork and tasks which may not always suit our way of working.

When choosing a career or looking at the one you have, consider the following;

• Are there any areas of the work which do not suit you?

• Does the job contain tasks which you know you will have difficulty with?

• If you face any difficulties, could there be solutions?

• Will your choice of career play on your strengths?

• Is it a flexible career, so that you can change route if you face any difficulties?

Learning Can Be Fun with Phonics
Sue Briggs

'**Phonics**' should not be a 'mind numbing collection of worksheets assigned by teachers to keep pupils busy!' (Adams, 1990). In the National Literacy Strategy, U.K., there is heavy stress on learning to read and spell using one sensory area e.g., 'phonics' (an auditory exercise) or 'whole words' e.g. 'sight words' (a visual exercise). Children with dyslexia do not learn to read and spell easily as the memory in one or both of these sensory areas is not working as efficiently as the others.

Successful learning takes place when all the sensory areas (visual, auditory, tactile, kinaesthetic) interact simultaneously. Children with dyslexia learn successfully in an active way by hearing, seeing, repeating and saying aloud, doing and playing. They need to develop their learning skills in a different way e.g. by using a structured multisensory approach so the stronger senses can be used while also exercising the weaker areas. We can make learning to read and spell fun with games and activities that develop and reinforce these learning skills, in school and at home (Briggs, 1999).

Developing phonological awareness. There are several stages which can be introduced with games and activities from 2 years. Older children who have not succeeded with reading and spelling should be taken through the earlier stages to see where they may have a learning gap.

1. Listening is an active skill

It requires children to focus their attention, concentrate, discriminate and hold a sequence of sounds in memory. Games can be played, at home and in school to improve each of these skills. Games such as the following:

- 'What sounds can be heard, in the room, outside, or even internally?'

- 'What sounds are comforting or worrying, loud or quiet?'

- Can sounds of animals etc. from a tape be identified?

- Play 'Chinese Whispers' and listen to a whispered message, the last child repeating what they think they have heard.

- Can they remember a sequence of sounds or use pictures to order sounds heard on a tape?'

2. Rhyme

Children can listen, sing and learn Nursery Rhymes.

- Can they choose a toy from a basket, name it and give a word that rhymes with it?

- Can they make up silly rhyming sentences or give the missing word?

- Play rhyming catch or hopscotch.

- Use singing rhyme games and number counting rhymes to detect rhyme and rhythm?

3. Syllable Segmentation.

Tapping out syllables in words from 3 years, can be fun when made into a game. These games are valuable exercises for language development and for naming and retrieving words from memory:

- Tap syllables in names of toys using parts of the body or using musical instruments.

- Use a bag to feel and guess the object.

- Make a board game.

4. Onset and Rime - the next stage.

Children, by 4 years, find it easier to separate words into units (or chunks) of sounds e.g. 'st -a- mp' before segmenting words into phonemes. They become familiar with the Beginning, Middle and End (BME) of words. The end of a word is called the 'rime' e.g. '- in' when the last letters are the same. The beginning letters are 'onset' letters e.g. 't' -in, 'p' - in, 'sp' -in.

Collect toys or draw pictures of objects with similar rimes.

Can they find pictures with words in common discovering the rime?

Find the odd pictures which do not rime. What is different?

Make sets of cards with onset and rime. Play matching games or three of a kind, snap, pairs and Bingo. All these games are played before sound symbols are introduced e.g. phonemes.

5. Initial Sound Games - Introduce sorting games.

Use toys with the same sounds at the beginning of the words. Draw objects on cards and ask the children to give the initial sound. When the initial letter has been introduced, play matching games, post boxes, Bingo or fishing games using magnets.

Play 'Kim's Game' putting several objects on a tray to be identified and then cover the tray. How many objects have the same initial sound? Cover the tray and remove an object. Ask the children to name the object which has been removed. Ask what tactics have they used to remember in each exercise. It is important that children become aware of learning and memory strengths as this also raises self-esteem and confidence. Later use the final sounds in words. Medial vowel sounds are difficult to identify for children with an auditory difficulty.

6. Crack the Code 1

Sequencing the Alphabet is a separate exercise with wooden capital letters. They provide valuable tactile - kinaesthetic experience and are less confusing, easier to identify and name, and reversals can be avoided. Teach the alphabet letter names in sequences of three (except for 'VW'). Put the letters into a cloth bag and in turn, the children name the first letter they touch before withdrawing it. They win the letter if it is named correctly. At a later stage they learn to match lower case letters to upper case letters.

7. Crack the Code 2

SMART Memory Cue Cards are introduced at the same time. The cue cards help children with dyslexia to develop an automatic response to sounds and their spellings. These high frequency letters are referred to (Briggs, 1999) as the 's a n d p i t' letters. Each phoneme is introduced step by step using the structured order of high frequency letters in words. The children draw their picture for the cue word on the reverse of the card when they have their own individual cards, or if used as a class exercise, a picture is drawn on A4 cards. The picture is the visual cue to the sound of the phoneme. If children have been taught correctly, the **visual memory** is triggered as they **give the cue word first** and **the sound heard** while looking at the symbol on the face of the card. They collect more 'memory' cards when they can give quick responses.

8. A structured multisensory approach

This means that **whole language** can be used from the beginning as words can be made and put into simple sentences for illustrated stories using punctuation. Learning can be active with games which reinforce and improve skills by linking sounds in words for reading and spelling.

Children with dyslexia, or in mainstream classes in the UK and in International Schools, are always keen to see how many words can be made with the 's a n d p i t' letters. Accepting the challenge, 'Year 6' in one International School, made 126 words using the two short vowel sounds. They searched through dictionaries, the thesaurus and the Internet. They wrote and illustrated stories on computers for children in younger classes. They devised card and board games, made quizzes and crosswords - and they had fun!

Teachers, parents and children agree internationally, that by playing games they have not only made progress in 'phonics' but have also joined a world wide club in learning to overcome many reading and spelling difficulties in a fun way.

Copyright 'Learning Can Be Fun' © by Suzanne Briggs, 1999. A set of three structured language games books published by Egon Publishers.

E-mail: suxmex@yahoo.com

'Beginning to Read' by M. J. Adams (1990). Materials also available from LDA Publishers.

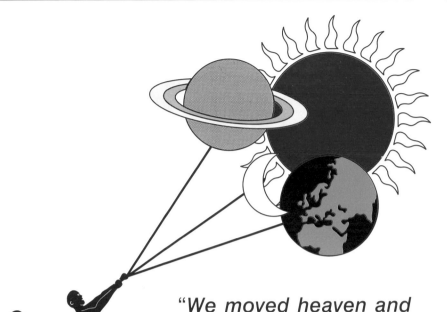

"We moved heaven and earth to get our child into Northease Manor School..."

Dyslexia presents huge problems.

Northease specialises in solving them.

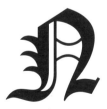

Ring the Secretary 01273 472915
e-mail: northease@msn.com
or fax: 01273 472202
(Lewes, East Sussex)

DfEE Recognised – CRESTED Category A
Amongst Top Ten Special Schools HMCI (1996)

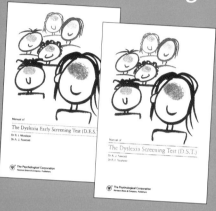
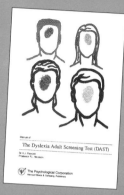
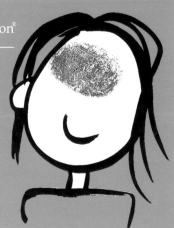

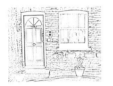

Parents of Dyslexic Children - Responsibilities and Opportunities

Carol Orton takes a look at the what parents need to know, and how best to use that information.

1996 Education Act

Educational professionals all agree, at least in theory, that wherever possible, parents must be fully involved in their child's education. Where a child has special educational needs this is especially important.

Parents should be pro-active in making sure that their child's learning difficulties are being properly addressed. Their concerns should be taken seriously and investigated.

Parents' responsibilities

"The parent of every child of compulsory school age shall cause him to receive efficient full-time education suitable -

a) to his age, ability and aptitude, and

b) to any special educational needs he may have, either by regular attendance at school or otherwise."

Section 7, 1996 Act

The Code of Practice

The 1996 Education Act says there must be a Code of Practice which gives practical guidance to local education authorities (LEAs) and school governing bodies on their responsibilities towards all children with special educational needs. The Code strongly emphasises the value of partnership with parents. It is the duty of LEAs and school governors to "have regard to the provisions of the code." They must not ignore it. A new Code of Practice will be published in the Spring of 2001 and will come into force later in the year.

Copies of the existing Code and the new draft can be obtained by ringing DfEE Publications on 0845 602 2260 or emailing dfee@prologistics.co.uk

Section 317 of the 1996 Education Act says that governors must do their best to secure the right sort of help for children with SEN. It is expected that schools will provide support for most children with SEN. Only a tiny minority will have SEN so severe that they cannot be met by the school. The Code says that the importance of early identification, assessment and provision for any child who may have SEN cannot be over-emphasised so parents should not be fobbed off when they suspect their child may be dyslexic.

Parents have a right to information in the form of the school's SEN Policy, which has to contain specific details about

- how the school organises special educational provision

- how the school allocates resources to pupils with special educational needs

- how the governors evaluate the success of the education given to children with special educational needs.

Every school will have a Special Educational Needs Co-ordinator (SENCo) who is responsible for the day to day co-ordination and management of the extra help that children with special educational needs require.

The governors' annual report to parents must also include specific information about the SEN policy, including the way resources have been allocated.

Statutory Assessment of Special Educational Needs

The needs of the great majority of children who have special educational needs should be met effectively by the school. However where they are not, the LEA should make a "statutory assessment" of the child's needs. Before making the assessment the LEAs must tell parents of their right to make representations and submit written evidence. Parents have a right, under Section 329 of the 1996 Education Act, to request that the LEA carries out such an assessment.

Parents are strongly advised to seek advice from their local dyslexia association before they start this process.

Parents have a right to put in their own report and their independent expert's advice. There are time limits for each stage of the assessment process and regulations about who should contribute. These are described in the Code of Practice.

Statements of Special Educational Needs

If, after completing the assessment, the LEA decides it needs to make a statement they must first send parents a 'proposed statement'. Parents may 'make representations' about the statement if they disagree with any part of it and may request a meeting to discuss the statement, which the LEA must arrange. The BDA suggests parents contact their local dyslexia association for help as soon as they receive a 'proposed statement'.

The statement itself must describe all the child's needs and provision to meet each and every one of them. The BDA has produced a leaflet, Analysing a statement, obtainable via the Helpline, 0118 966 8271 or the BDA's website www.bda-dyslexia.org.uk/

Once the LEA has made a statement it is responsible for

arranging the provision even if they have delegated the money to the schools.

Annual Review

The LEA must review a statement at least once a year. There is a strict procedure which must be followed. This allows parents plenty of notice of the review meeting and invites them to give written advice. Again the BDA suggests parents contact their local dyslexia association for help as soon as they receive a letter about their child's annual review.

If the LEA is thinking about 'ceasing to maintain' the statement they should only do so after close consultation with parents.

The Special Educational Needs Tribunal

Parents may appeal to the Special Educational Needs Tribunal if the LEA:

- Refuses to assess
- Refuses to make a statement after an assessment
- Ceases to maintain a statement

and

- if parents disagree with the contents of a statement.

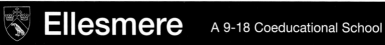
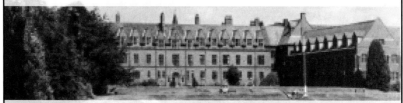
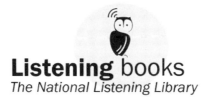

Thinking and planning to meet special needs: The importance of the IEP

Carol Orton, BDA policy and information manager explains the crucial role of individual education plans in enabling a dyslexic child to succeed at school.

Individual Education Plans (IEPs) are management documents, identifying provision to match needs and setting targets to evaluate success. They are not lesson plans and they do not have to be lengthy, time-consuming documents. The new draft Code of Practice suggests they should be 'crisp'. Nevertheless the most important part of an IEP is the thinking and planning.

Thinking

- What is this child finding so hard to learn?

- Why is he or she having such problems?

- Do I understand the way he learns?

Planning

- What can I do to make her learn better?

- Why have I chosen that approach?

- Who will deliver it? How often? Where?

Targets

- What do I expect him to achieve as a result of this extra help?

- How will I know if she has learnt effectively?

- How can I explain to all his teachers so they understand why she finds some things so difficult?

Review

- Is it working? If not, why not?

- Is she able to transfer her skills to the everyday curriculum?

- Do I really understand the way he learns?

- What can I do instead?   Something more? Something different?

- What needs to change in the classroom?

Children should be involved in developing and reviewing their IEPs. Dyslexic adults point to their understanding their own dyslexia as a major factor in being able to return to education and being successful in their careers. Dyslexic children, too, need to understand the way their dyslexia affects them and how they learn best. If they have the self-confidence to take control of their learning they are more likely to ask for help and build on that help.

Their questions may be

- What do I find difficult?

- How might I find it easier?

- If I learn best visually how can I apply this experience to French?

- How can I ask for help?

As well as a current IEP focusing on immediate short term targets, it is essential to develop an in-depth understanding of individual SEN, incorporating diagnostic information and evaluation of the child's response to different learning strategies.

It is a good idea to a maintain a SEN Profile running alongside his IEP, for background information. Its purpose matches Part 2 of a statement, described in case law as a 'diagnosis'. A thorough understanding of a child's SEN developed through his profile may prevent the need for a statement. It is especially useful as the child changes year groups or moves on to another school.

IEPs should be seen as an integral part of whole school planning. Wherever possible whole school policies should address at least some aspects of classroom working that children with SEN find difficult. Moreover evaluations of SEN provision, from IEP reviews, should inform whole school planning.

However most dyslexic children will continue to need the oversight and planning associated with the new School Action element of the new Code of Practice.

Children do not grow out of their dyslexia. Their problems are not solved when they learn to read or to type. Once they have learnt to read, they need to read to learn and different skills are required. Decoding is a very different process to assimilating knowledge. Remembering a few more spellings is very different from demonstrating knowledge and understanding. The new Code aims to enable pupils with special educational needs to reach their full potential, to be fully included in their school communities and make a successful transition to adulthood. Weaknesses in short term memory, speed of information processing and organisation must all be addressed if the dyslexic child is to become a successful independent learner.

Ten ways of becoming a partner in your child's education

Planning, organisation and studying are not only a key part of learning for dyslexic students, but also integral in the support procedure for parents. Carol Orton tell how.

- Find out as much as you can about your child's dyslexia. Read some books about dyslexia. Join your local dyslexia association where you can talk to other parents and dyslexia specialists.

- Become familiar with The Code of Practice on the Identification and Assessment of Special Educational Needs. Get one free from the Department for Education and Employment's publication centre by ringing 0845 602 2260.

- Be as clear as possible just what difficulties you think your child has and why you are worried. Dyslexic children have obvious difficulties with reading and spelling. But these are symptoms of underlying difficulties with memory, phonological awareness and information processing. Articles in this handbook will help you understand the effect these will have on his or her learning.

- Describe your child's difficulties in detail. Take reading as an example. What happens when he can't read a word? Does he guess wildly? Does he attempt to work it out? How successfully? In continuous reading does he make errors? e.g. miss words? syllables? (beginning, middle, end) Can he read for information, a bus timetable, a computer game manual or the TV Times? Does he seem to be concentrating so hard on sounding words out, or read so slowly, that he can't remember what he has read? Can he remember/understand a sentence/ page/chapter? What strategies does he use to avoid reading? What help does he need? What works at home, if anything? e.g. "If I read the text book to him he can do the homework."

- The 'dyslexia stick man' is a reminder of the range of difficulties with which a dyslexic child may have problems. Describe each of your child's difficulties. Don't rely on your other people's evidence to speak for you. Use it instead to back up what you say. Examples of a child's work are useful evidence.

- Think carefully about the help he needs and why. If you are seeking a statutory assessment you must show why his local school cannot provide it. Remember that you are describing a 'difficulty in learning' or a disability that 'prevents or hinders' your child from making use of educational facilities, not simply his scores on certain tests (Section 312, 1996 Education Act).

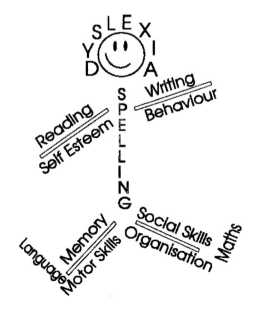

- Keep a ring binder file with all reports and correspondence, in date order. Don't be tempted to stuff it all in a drawer! Try and keep notes of all telephone calls. Send letters to confirm in writing what has been said at meetings and on the phone - keep copies.

- Keep a diary about the day to day happenings at school and at home if you need to illustrate the difficulties your child is having. Make notes of the things your child says about his problems.

- Prepare for meetings - the focus should be your child. It is very easy to get distracted into an argument about who said what and when, or delays in procedures, and then find you have not said anything that really worries you about how difficult your child is finding everything. It is a good idea to send a letter saying what you want to discuss at the meeting beforehand. Give the school copies of any evidence you have in advance. If at all possible, take someone with you to make sure that the people at the meeting stick to the point. The other person migh also take notes. Try and stay calm. Getting angry or upset really doesn't help. Send a letter afterwards confirming what was said.

- Keep encouraging your child and show him or her that you really love them. Home is somewhere he should be safe and happy, however hard he finds things at school. Try and keep your frustrations with schools and LEAs to yourself.

And finally, allow yourself to escape from the pressures sometimes.

Some really useful ways that parents can help

Jane Jacobson review how parents may help their dyslexic childand ensure a balanced approach to the help provided.

Explain dyslexia to your child

You may think this is so basic that it doesn't need to be mentioned, but sometimes the obvious can be overlooked.

No fault, no blame: emphasise that the problems s/he has been experiencing are not his/her fault - children can easily believe that they are to blame because they must be doing something wrong. (By the way, this goes for you too - let yourself off the hook).

Focus on differences rather than difficulties: explain how dyslexic people learn in a different way and therefore need to be taught in different ways - that is why they may need some special separate lessons

Accentuate the positive: everyone has their strong and weak points - find your child's strengths and encourage them to develop. Point to some good role models - for example Steve Redgrave, Benjamin Zephaniah, Whoopi Goldberg.

Tell it how it is: there's no getting away from the fact that dyslexic children need to work harder than their non-dyslexic peers to achieve their best at school - dyslexic children need to know this, but at the same time they should be encouraged to think about their future successes.

Resources:

So, you think you've got problems? Birkett, R. Egon Publishers Ltd. (1993)

Let's Discuss Dyslexia. Sanders, P & Myers S. Watts Books. (1995)

Keep a balanced approach

You will already know that you need to keep on this problem - if you sit back and expect school to do everything you will not be addressing many of the difficulties your child needs to overcome to succeed in later life. On the other hand, blind panic would be equally unproductive and could do permanent damage to your relationship with your child. Try to strike a happy medium:

Encouragement not pressure: it will be hard enough for your child to keep up at school - they need to be encouraged every step of the way and helped to believe in themselves.

Praise not criticism: this comes back to accentuating the positive. There are many ways to praise what a child has done well without homing in on the mistakes.

Relationship with school: whatever you think of your child's school and teachers, try to keep it to yourself. Their job will be made that much harder if your child has lost respect for them.

By the way - keeping a balanced approach will help save your sanity, too!

Teach your child to touch type

Most children are both confident and competent when it comes to computers. Your dyslexic child will probably come to depend a great deal on computers for note taking, revision, essay writing and even in some cases for exams. It will really make a difference if they can touch type. There are several programmes on the market for self learning, but if you can, find a course such as Touch Type Read & Spell.

Resources

LDA computer coordinator - look up your local dyslexia association in the blue pages of this book - the computer coordinator will be able to give you information about different programmes and also about courses in your area.

Help make reading fun

If your child is struggling with learning to read, the chances are that reading books are the least fun thing s/he can think of. They may also feel belittled if the sorts of books they are able to read are written for a much younger reader. Try the following to make reading fun:

High interest books: there are now many 'high interest, low reading age' books on the market. These stories have an appropriate content for older children but are written in language they can cope with. Try your local library, or call your local dyslexia association for more information.

Recorded stories: this is a great way for your child to enjoy the stories others can read for themselves, without the struggle. For younger children there are audio tapes available with reading books to read and listen at the same time. For others there is a wide range of audio tapes and, more frequently, CDs.

Resources

Seven Ways to Help Your Child With Reading. Geere, B.

The Listening Books - see handbook advert page 186

For books for reluctant readers
    www.barringtonstoke.co.uk
    www.booktrust.org.uk/reluctant.html
    www.puffin.co.uk/library/lib_3.html

Help your child acquire some study skills

Most children benefit from learning how to learn, and this is especially true of dyslexics. 'Study skills' covers a wide range of activities such as note taking, speed reading, essay writing, memory techniques, effective revision and more. The best way to learn study skills is to do a course - find out about study skills courses from this handbook and from your local dyslexia association. If this is not possible, however, below are some self help resources. Also see the article on page 268 by Christine Ostler on Study Skills.

Mind maps are particularly useful and fun - I use them myself to 'brainstorm' and organise ideas. They don't have to be works of art and are easy to do - older dyslexics will find it extremely helpful to learn this skill. As an alternative to hand drawn you could try the computerised version, Inspiration. (See the article on page 262 by Andi Sanderson.)

Resources

Use Your Head. Buzan, T. BBC (1989)

Get Ahead (Video). Israel, L & Buzan, T. Island World Video (1992).

Learn How To Study - A Realistic Approach. Rowntree, D. Warner Books (1998)

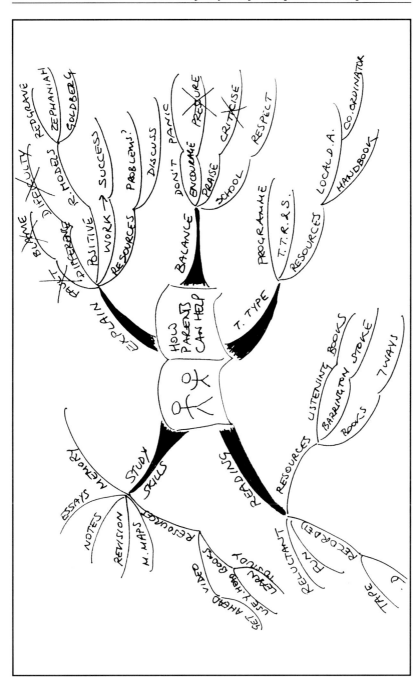

Using Inspiration

Inspiration is a piece of computer software which works with the visual talents of many dyslexics. Basically it is a visual mapping tool which supports the often random, chaotic and disorganised thoughts of dyslexics allowing such thoughts to be captured, restructured and presented in a visual manner. Here Andi Sanderson explains how to use it.

Inspiration enables the users to create a visual map of ideas in much the same way as Tony Buzan's 'Mind Mapping'® concept, creating a diagram such as:-

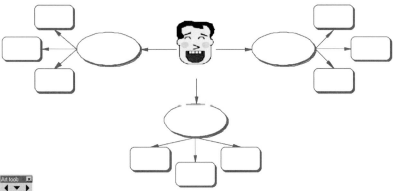

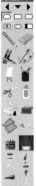

The software includes its own library of 1,250 (Version 6) shapes and pictures which is located on a palette on the left hand side of the screen.

All shapes and pictures in the Inspiration library can be coloured in a variety of colour schemes making each concept map unique and individual, and sufficiently flexible to express the ideas of the users.

Hence a simple picture of shape can be transformed by colour to reflect subtleties in ideas.

Text can be added at anytime to either symbols and pictures or along adjoining arrows and lines, in a range of fonts, sizes and colours. In the latest version of Inspiration (Version 6) a spell checker assists the dyslexic in producing text.

Along the top of the page is a simple tool bar allowing easy access to the many facilities that Inspiration supports. Three of the most useful tools besides the Spell Checker, are 'Create keys', 'Arrange' and 'Outline':

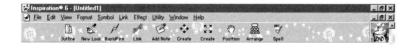

Create Keys

These keys are used to 'create' further symbols etc. The tips of each directional arrow turn blue as the cursor runs over it – when the directional arrow turns blue a left click of the mouse will create another base symbol – which can be changed by selecting from the symbol and/or colour pallets.

Arrange

The 'arrange' key is used to restructure diagrams into a more orderly and equidistant design. Hence something which looks a little unprofessional can be transformed into a very smart visual diagram ! For example changing this:-

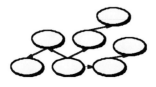
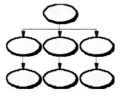

Outline

Inspiration has the facility to turn, for example, a flow chart into text format which can be copied and pasted into any other application to compliment and enhance work prepared elsewhere, such as Word. Indeed when in the 'Outline' application, additional thoughts can be added in words which automatically appear in diagrammatic form when switched to that outline. In this respect Inspiration also appeals to those word based thinkers who can use Inspiration to turn linear text into a pictorial and very visual format.

Templates/Guides

Some 35 different templates can be selected and added to, or indeed altered as required. These help those who find starting difficult: they can build impressive visual maps representing their ideas in a relatively painless way. Inspiration also produces guides for teachers in order that it can be used effectively not only as a general tool in the classroom but also to compliment and enhance the delivery of the National Curriculum. Titles include:-

- Meeting Standards with Inspiration
- Classroom Ideas Using Inspiration: For Teachers by Teachers

'Classroom ideas Using Inspiration' includes lesson suggestions for:-

- Brainstorming techniques
- Concept mapping in science
- Designing a web page and other multimedia projects
- Understanding stories using graphic organizers
- Analysing events using the 'Outline' view

Who is it for ?

Inspiration can be used by a number of age groups as it is easy to learn and simple to use. Many are able to grasp the basics within minutes. Thus 5 year olds are able to create simple outlines such as a diagram of their family and post graduate students are able to construct intricate flow charts or perhaps a chain of complex chemical reactions.

It is also very useful for anyone struggling to organise their thoughts for assignments or an essay, as ideas can be quickly transferred to the screen. When on the screen ideas can be organised, regrouped and transferred into a necessary linear text form via the outline tool and used as a plan to guide their writing.

In essence Inspiration provides the dyslexic with a degree of independence so often desired and seldom experienced. Inspiration offers the means of bringing the non word thoughts locked inside the creative part of a dyslexic brain to life whether it be a simple flow chart or a clear representation of complex relationships. It enables the user to organise random thoughts and bursts of inspiration into a logical form which can be used to reflect suppressed talent and unknown ability.

Trial Version

For those who would like to try before they buy – it is possible to download a trial version of Inspiration from their web site at www.inspiration.com or iANSYST's site at www.dyslexic.com/inspir.htm.

Inspiration Version 6 is available from iANSYST (see address and contact details below) and costs £90 + VAT for a single user licence, £59.95 + VAT if you are a teacher or student. To use Inspiration you will need Windows 95, 98, ME, NT4 or 2000 plus 8mb of RAM. There is also an Inspiration MAC version which costs the same as the PC version.

A colour printer is very useful when using Inspiration.

iANSYST Training Products

The White House

72 Fen Road

Cambridge

CB4 1UN

Tel: 01223 42 01 01

Fax 01223 42 66 44

Email: sales@dyslexic.com

www.dyslexic.com

For discussions on the use of mind maps see the articles by Jane Jacobson (page 257) and Andi Sanderson (page 262)

Study Skills: using strengths and weaknesses

The key to successful studying is to recognise your strengths and weaknesses. Make the most of your strengths, but don't fight your weaknesses. Rather, make them work for you. Christine Ostler tell you how.

1. Are you disorganised, forgetful, poor at time-management?

Good! It probably means that you are innovative, creative and not bound by the constraints of left-brained, sequential, logical thinking. However, to be able to use your lateral thinking talents to the full, some organisational skills will be needed. Try some of the following:

- Keep small notebooks, with pencils attached, scattered around the house and in your pocket so that you can jot down ideas as they come to you.

- A mini-cassette recorder could be used instead of notebooks.

- Use a large year-planner pinned up somewhere prominent so that you can monitor the passing of time and can plan ahead. Fill in module deadlines or exams, fieldtrips, holidays and your birthday (you won't be spending hours on your homework that day, so you must make sure you get ahead earlier in the week!).

- Use a diary – depending on your circumstances, this could be pocket-sized, a more elaborate personal organiser (mine is A5 and includes plastic wallets into which I slip letters and memos that need attention), an electronic palmtop organiser or a homework diary supplied by your school. The important thing is to use it daily and not to rely on your memory.

- Use a check-list at the beginning of the term to ensure that you have all the equipment you need.

- Make five copies of your school timetable: keep one in your pocket, one in your pencil case, one stuck to the inside of your school locker, pin one up at home and refer to it before setting off for school each day to check what you are going to need, and give the fifth one to a responsible adult or friend for when you've lost the other four! (Be honest, you know this can happen!)

2. Do you find it difficult getting started on your homework?

Think of it as a workout – Warm up - Work hard - Cool down

- Warm up

- Read through the instructions or questions

- Look at notes made in class

- Look at previous examples

- Look at your textbook

- Ask yourself, "What do I have to do? How am I going to do it?"

- Link this new task to what you already know

- Work hard

- Set yourself a time limit

- Promise yourself a reward for when you are finished

- Now get on!

- Cool down

- Read/look through what you have done

- Read the instructions/questions again

- Ask yourself, "Have I finished?"

- If "Yes", check for accuracy

- If "No", what else needs to be done? When will you finish?

3. Does your mind wander when reading?

Try some of these strategies:

- Highlight key words

- Use 'Highlighters' (repositionable adhesive highlighting index tabs made by Snopake) if it's not your own book

- Write yourself questions after each paragraph

- Make notes[1]: numbered points, a mindmap[2] or flowchart

- Draw pictures to illustrate main points

- Read aloud

4. When writing an essay do ideas flood into your mind in random order so that you don't know where to start?

- Write each idea onto a small piece of paper

- Spread the pieces out in front of you

- Group connected ideas – these will form paragraphs

- Discard ideas that do not relate to the title of the essay or coursework

- Decide on the main point for each pile of paper

- Arrange these piles into a logical sequence

- Write a topic sentence for each pile – this will introduce or sum up what the paragraph is about

- Add supporting detail which you have listed on the other pieces of paper in each pile – one idea per sentence

- This will give you the body of the essay – you may need to add a general introduction and a conclusion

Alternatively, plan your essay using a Mindmap™.

- Take a plain piece of paper and place it 'landscape'.

- Write your title in the centre of the page.

- Decide on the main points you wish to make – draw a branch for each point radiating from your title.

- Draw smaller branches from each main branch listing your supporting detail.

- Include an introduction which will give an overview of what you are going to write about.

- Finish with a conclusion that will pull all of the threads together – you may be required to give an opinion or to evaluate how successful you feel that you have been in addressing the task.

- Number the branches in the order in which you will write them up.

- Watch the 'Get Ahead' video to see how to make a mindmap.

5. Do you find learning for tests difficult?

Before you start:

- Check that you are clear about what you have to learn (if in doubt, telephone a friend).

- Check how you will be tested – one-word answers, writing a paragraph/essay, multi-choice, labelling a diagram, orally etc.

- Is spelling accuracy essential or is legibility sufficient?

- Are you permitted to use a calculator?

- Do you understand what it is you are trying to learn? If 'no', read around the subject, consult a revision book, ask a friend.

Make sure that you keep active – (see note 3)

- Use Look – Say – Cover – Write – Check not only for learning spellings but for learning formulae, people's names and what they did, the order of biological functions (e.g. respiration), etc.

- Use small strips of Post-it notes to cover the labels on diagrams. Number these strips and then make a numbered list of what the labels should say. Remove Post-its and check.

- Record questions and answers onto cassette tape. When playing back the tape, use the pause button to say the answer before you hear it.

- Revise with a friend – test each other.

- Transfer notes onto a mindmap. Pin onto your bedroom wall and study for a few minutes before going to sleep each evening.

6. Be creative

Identify the areas you find difficult or which stop you from being an efficient student and experiment with different strategies. There is no right way or wrong way to study, but there is a way that will work for you. You will have good days, and not so good days. Try to work out what made the good day 'good' and use that approach again. Happy studying!

Notes

1 and 3. Ostler C. Study Skills – a Pupil's Survival Guide Ammonite Books (p. 29)

2. Get Ahead –   video with Lana Israel available from The Buzan Centre, 54 Parkstone Road, Poole, Dorset BH15 2PX

Inspiration – MindMapping© CDRom

Christine Ostler is Director of the Susan Hampshire Centre at Cobham Hall – author of 'Study Skills: a Pupil's Survival Guide' and 'Dyslexia: a Parents' Survival Guide'. She also has in preparation (with Frances Ward), 'Advanced Study Skills: a Student's Survival Guide for AS, A Level and Advanced GNVQ'.

Part 4 - Around dyslexia

This section contains chapters on other conditions which in some cases are found to occur together with dyslexia.

Part 4 - Around dyslexia

Double diagnosis or developmental diversity

Dyslexia and dyspraxia often occur together, and in any checklist for dyslexia you will often find descriptors which some would say are dyspraxia. So what is the difference? Here, Gail Goedkoop, former director of the Helen Arkell Dyslexia Centre, looks at some of the difficulties of separating out the two.

Many parents bring their child for an assessment in order to answer the question is he dyslexic or not? But lately more parents have been coming with the question, is he dyslexic or dyspraxic,or maybe ADHD? A problem can arise after assessment, if parents feel their question has not been answered. Parents may be asking these questions for two reasons: 1) they believe a label is necessary to get the correct action for their child, 2) media articles and some books can make it appear that diagnosis to a label is quite clear cut.

The fact is that although the proliferation of labels for varieties of specific learning difficulties has alerted parent and teachers alike to the wide variety of problems beyond reading, the mere application of a label may not result in the correct remedial action. For example, many dyslexics need training to hear sounds within words, but a dyslexic who spells phonetically probably will not need training to hear sounds within words, but a dyslexic who spells phonetically probably will not need such a training programme. There is a worrying trend in over-stretched schools these days to just pull out a popular remedial programme for the Learning Support Assistant to deliver, without considering its appropriateness for the particular child.

A second worry is that the individuality of the child may be

Similarities between dyslexia and dyspraxia

Commonly used descriptors of both SpLDs

Late development of speech

Difficulties with speech

Problems with self-dressing

Confused laterality

Forgetful/memory problems

Difficulty following instructions/directions

Poor sense of direction

Problems with orientation

Problems with sequencing

Poor organisation/untidy

Poor processing of verbal information

Sometimes clumsy

Difficulty copying from blackboard

Odd pencil grip

Poor handwriting

Difficulty getting it down on paper

Inconsistent school performance

Difficulty paying attention

Anxious

Sensitive

Low self-esteem

obscured by the application of a label particularly with the 'dys' syllable encouraging us to ignore strengths, talents, interests and compensation strategies.

To complicate matters further, the rather unfortunate term co-morbidity is used to describe the situation where an individual appears to have the symptoms of more than one condition - a double diagnosis. Again such a term discourages us from appreciating all the positive traits of an individual, but the fact remains that there is indeed a great overlap between the various SpLD profiles, perhaps as much as 40% between dyslexia and dyspraxia, and between dyslexia and ADD.

Because parents ask for labels, assessors tend to try to provide them, but an excellent solution to the labels dilemma is Dr Melvin Levine's model of Neurodevelopmental Diversity. He proposes the following parameters of learning: Attention, Memory, Language, Temporal-Sequential Ordering, Spatial Ordering, neuromotor Function, Higher Order Cognition, Social Cognition. Each parameter is considered in terms of the many subskills involved, whose strengths and dysfunctions combined can create a myriad of individual patterns. (Wide variations exists between individuals, and differences need not represent pathology or abnormality.) Levine's assessment model is embodied in the PEEX and PEERAMID assessment batteries which generate a highly detailed profile of a child in terms of a wide variety of subskills. Such a profile leads easily into an appropriate individualised prescription and management programme. Management by profile must include the following 5 essential elements.

1) Intervention at the Breakdown Points - specific weaknesses are identified by task analysis, and teaching activities designed to strengthen the weak subskills.

2) Consideration of additional supports - for example, parent support, speech and language therapy, occupational therapy, counselling, social skills training.

Dyslexia - dyspraxia contrasted

DYSPRAXIA	DYSLEXIA
Late motor development	Early or normal motor milestones
Weak posture and muscle tone	
Verbal IQ> Performance IQ (almost always)	Performance IQ > Verbal IQ (often)
Poor gross motor skills, poor at PE	Often good at sports
Poor fine motor skills, dislike of crafts and art	Strengths in art and craft skills
Difficulty with social skills	Often strong in personal skills
Usually no reading difficulty unless visual reading problems	Usually reading problems
	Problems with word finding, rhymes, phonological awareness
More writing than spelling difficulty	Always spelling problems
Weak at Maths concepts	Often good at Maths concepts
More likely a difficult birth history	More often genetic history
	by Gail Goedkoop, HADC

3) By-pass Strategies - for example, alternative ways to demonstrate knowledge, word-processing and IT support, adjustment to curriculum load. Such allowances must be combined with 'humiliation protection'.

4) Strengthening the Strengths - talents and enthusiasms are identified, and opportunities sought for these to develop, flourish, and be recognised and valued.

5) De-mystification - students must be given the conceptual framework and vocabulary to discuss and understand their own individual profile. This leads to acceptance and active participation in the management programme which ultimately can lead to self-esteem, self-advocacy, and personal success.

Of the 5, de-mystification is of primary importance, and a prerequisite to the success of all the other programme components, as it enables the child to value his differences and uniqueness.

Books and material by Dr Melvin Levine, published by Educator's Publishing Company are available from the Helen Arkell Dyslexia Centre.

Educational Care (for teachers and psychologists)

All kinds of Minds (for primary aged children for de-mystification)

Keeping Ahead in School (for secondary aged students for de-mystification)

PEEX - assessment battery ages 6-9 (for trained specialist teachers and psychologists)

PEERAMID - assessment battery ages 9-16 (for specialist teachers and psychologists)

Dyscalculia: Another specific learning difficulty?

Dr Steve Chinn, principal of Mark College and a leading authority of dyslexia and maths, looks at the evidence for considering maths difficulty as a separate difficulty from dyslexia.

There are several aspects of this topic which I would like to explore. It makes sense to begin by looking at some of the definitions of dyscalculia.

Developmental dyscalculia is defined by Bakwin (1960) as a 'difficulty with counting' and by Cohn (1968) as a 'failure to recognise numbers or manipulate them in an advanced culture'. Gerstmann (1957) describes dyscalculia (Gerstmann's syndrome) as 'an isolated disability to perform simple or complex arithmetical operations and an impairment of orientation in the sequence of numbers and their fractions'

Various sources

Developmental dyscalculia is a structural disorder of mathematical abilities which has its origin in a genetic or congenital disorder of those parts of the brain that are the direct anatomico-physiological substrate of the maturation of the mathematical abilities adequate to age, without a simultaneous disorder of general mental functions.

Kosc 1970

The word 'dyscalculia' means difficulty performing math calculations. In other words, it just means 'math difficulty' and specifically it means a learning disability which affects math.

The term is seldom used within public schools (USA) because of the lack of any strict or measurable criteria.

The Internet

Difficulty in mathematics is the low achievement of a person on a certain occasion which manifests itself as performance below standard of the age-group of this person or below his own abilities as a consequence of inadequate cognitive, affective, volitional, motor or sensory etc development. The cause for inadequate development may be of various kinds.

Magne (1978)

Dyscalculia refers to a disorder in the ability to do or to learn mathematics, ie, difficulty in number conceptualisation, understanding number relationships and difficulty in learning algorithms (procedures) and applying them. (An irregular impairment of ability).

Sharma (1990)

These definitions, with the possible exception of Kosc's, define dyscalculia as a lower achievement in mathematics than would be expected from general ability, a specific learning difficulty in mathematics. From my experience of over thirty years of teaching, difficulties in maths are not rare, but how many qualify as dyscalculia is a hard question to answer.

There are many reasons why pupils may underachieve in maths. It could be difficulty in memorising and recalling basic facts. It could be that the unique language of maths causes problems. It could be that the learning style of the pupil did not match the learning style of the teacher. It could be that a teacher's own anxieties about maths transfer to the pupil. It could be that the culture of maths requires pupils to work quickly (look in the Numeracy Strategy to see how often speed words such as 'rapidly, quickly' occur).

There is little in the research literature about dyscalculia. There is a little more on the difficulties with maths experienced by dyslexic pupils. So my next point is to consider a possible connection between dyscalculia and dyslexia.

As a comparison to dyslexia where, incidentally definitions are increasingly focusing solely on language difficulties, the learning and doing of maths is quite different to learning and doing language. It is a very sequential, progressive subject, with new knowledge being dependent on previous learning. So for example, if a pupil has not realised that subtraction and addition are opposites, he might have difficulty with manipulating simple algebraic equations. Then, in maths the feedback from teachers is precise and based on 'right' or 'wrong'. In English, not many pupils get an essay 'wrong'. Judgment is more graded and usually avoids labelling work as 'wrong'. Spelling tests, of course, are an exception and may well contribute to the attitude problems with spelling. Most pupils try to avoid failure, especially recognised failure and may withdraw from involvement in the learning process. Again the sequential nature of maths exacerbates the consequences.

It happens that there are many learning characteristics of a dyslexic pupil that will also impact on maths. For example, Professor Miles uses two maths items in his Bangor Dyslexia test as part of the recognition of dyslexia in an individual. It has been my experience that dyslexic pupils usually have problems with maths, particularly with instant recall of times table facts. I would contend that difficulties in (at least some aspects of) maths are likely to accompany difficulties in language so, in this respect dyscalculia is frequently a difficulty occuring alongside dyslexia.

Does dyscalculia exist as a specific learning difficulty only with maths and not with language?

There is ample evidence to show extensive underachievement in maths, which resulted in the introduction of the Numeracy Strategy, but how much of this underachievement is due to dyscalculia is impossible to tell at this stage in our knowledge of the learning processes of maths.

As educators, we then have to decide, as with dyslexia, whether that difficulty is permanent and pervasive or responsive to appropriate remediation. My guess is, that in most cases, and if general intelligence is not impaired then truly significant improvements can be made. This also implies that some teaching can be inappropriate, as with dyslexia and that teaching may have had a crucial role in the development of an individual's difficulties with mathematics. This introduces my final point, the question of how much of the problem is inherent in the individual and how much is acquired as a result of inappropriate experiences.

As a teacher and an eternal optimist (the two should be comorbid) I believe virtually anyone can be taught some maths. I think attitude, anxiety and belief are critical factors and I believe that the range of teaching strategies used successfully with dyslexics will benefit dyscalculic pupils.

Developmental Verbal Dyspraxia

There are many difficulties associatied with dyslexia, including speech difficulties. Pam Williams takes a closer look at the problems of motor control that affect speech production.

What is it?

Dyspraxia refers to difficulties in achieving purposeful, sequential movement in the absence of muscular paresis (weakness). For children who present with developmental verbal dyspraxia, the movement difficulties primarily affect their ability to produce speech sounds and to sequence sounds together in words. In many cases, but not all, children with developmental verbal dyspraxia also have oro-motor dyspraxia affecting their ability to make and co-ordinate the movements of the larynx, lips, tongue and palate.

In the UK, the current favoured term is developmental verbal dyspraxia, recognising that the condition usually has both speech and language aspects. However, it is still sometimes referred to as articulatory dyspraxia and in the USA the condition is known as apraxia of speech.

For a parent or professional trying to understand the condition, a very useful definition of developmental verbal dyspraxia was provided by 13 year old Kevin who said "My mouth won't co-operate with my brain" (Stackhouse 1992a).

How do we recognise it?

Speech and language therapists usually diagnose currently by referring to checklists of characteristics and trying to identify a "symptom cluster" of presenting features. In addition to speech characteristics, checklists also usually refer to commonly reported language, learning, clinical and motor characteristics (Stackhouse 1992a).

The following list was produced by the Speech and Language Therapy department at the Nuffield Hearing and Speech Centre (1992):

Speech characteristics

- A limited range of consonant and vowel sounds
- Overuse of one sound ("favourite articulation")
- Vowel distortions
- Inconsistent production
- Breakdown in sequencing in words, particularly as they increase in length
- Errors of omission and substitution – idiosyncratic substitutions may occur
- Glottal stop insertions and substitutions
- Voice difficulties affecting volume, length, pitch, quality
- Resonance difficulties affecting the overall tone of the speech
- Prosodic difficulties affecting rate, rhythm, stress, intonation
- Unintelligible speech

Other co-occurring characteristics

- Family history of speech, language or literacy difficulties
- Delayed language development
- Delayed development of early speech skills eg babbling
- Feeding difficulties
- Oral dyspraxia affecting movements of the lips, tongue or palate
- Generalised developmental dyspraxia affecting fine and gross motor co-ordination

- Literacy difficulties affecting reading, spelling and writing
- Slow progress in therapy

One of the complicating issues in diagnosis is "the unfolding and changing nature of developmental verbal dyspraxia as a condition" (Stackhouse 1992b). The range of problems experienced unfold as the child progresses and more demands are placed upon him. Therefore the presentation of a child with developmental verbal dyspraxia is different at different ages and stages of development. Compare the following:

A young pre-school child may present with virtually no expressive speech, but the case history may give warning signs eg feeding difficulties, delayed early speech development, oral difficulties affecting the child's ability to blow, lick, suck, control dribbling etc.

For an older pre-school child who has already developed an amount of speech and language, there is likely to be an indicative pattern of speech errors as well as case history factors.

For the primary school-aged child, the speech may have improved greatly, with only subtle difficulties with complex long words remaining. However, difficulties with learning to read and spell have taken over as the main area of concern and are tell-tale signs of a "dyspraxic history".

Is there a relationship between developmental verbal dyspraxia and dyslexia?

Research has shown that children with developmental verbal dyspraxia whose speech difficulties persist beyond the age of 5.6 years are at risk of having literacy difficulties. The risk is increased if there is also a family history of speech, language or specific learning difficulties.

An impaired phonological processing system affects a child's ability to make sound and letter links and to carry out phonological awareness tasks essential for literacy acquisition. For many children, spelling tends to be affected more than reading.

What help do children with developmental verbal dyspraxia need?

Speech and language therapy

Referral should be made to a speech and language therapist, as early as possible, who will be able to assess the child, identify the presenting difficulties and advise on management of those difficulties.

Speech and language therapists may not necessarily assign a "label". Due to the complexity of diagnosis, therapists may prefer to be cautious and use more descriptive terminology eg "Ben has a significant speech disorder, characterised by dyspraxic features" rather than "Ben has developmental verbal dyspraxia".

It is generally recognised that children with developmental verbal dyspraxia do not get better without help. Ideally, they need access to direct speech and language therapy on a regular basis, supported by frequent practice outside the therapy sessions ie at home and/ or in school.

The Nuffield Dyspraxia Programme (1985; 1992; forthcoming) is one of the only published therapy approaches specifically for developmental verbal dyspraxia and is widely used by speech and language therapists in the UK and abroad. It offers a systematic approach to the assessment and treatment of developmental verbal dyspraxia and is particularly suitable for children aged 3-7 years. (Connery 1994)

Support in school

Although many children with developmental verbal dyspraxia attend mainstream school, they frequently require additional support on account of their speech and literacy difficulties, particularly in their early school years. Depending on their individual needs, this may be provided by special educational needs teachers and / or by learning support assistants.

A collaborative approach

Children with developmental verbal dyspraxia are best helped by a consistent, systematic approach to their difficulties. Communication and collaboration between all the professional involved is the best way to ensure this is provided.

References

Connery V.M. The Nuffield Dyspraxia Programme – working on the motor programming of speech. In: Before School: A handbook of approaches to intervention with pre-school language impaired children. Law J. (ed). London: AFASIC

Stackhouse J. (1992a) Developmental verbal dyspraxia: a longitudinal case study. In Campbell R, (ed) Mental Lives: Case studies in Cognition. Oxford: Blackwell.

Stackhouse J. (1992b) Developmental Verbal Dyspraxia I: A Review and Critique. European Disorders of Communication 27 (1) 19-34.

Pam Williams is Principal Speech and Language Therapist at the Nuffield Hearing and Speech Centre, RNTNE Hospital, Gray's Inn Road, London WC1N 8DA.For information on clinical services at the Nuffield Centre and the Nuffield Dyspraxia Centre Programme, please 'phone: 020-7915-1535

BOOK REVIEW

Reprinted from BDA Dyslexia Contact September 2000

Multilingualism, Literacy and Dyslexia - A Challenge for Educators

Lindsay Peer and Gavin Reid (editors)

David Fulton Publishers

2000, 290 pages, £19.50 including postage and handling

ISBN 1 85346 696 4

This fascinating book addresses a topic which, until recently, has been largely ignored. Lindsay Peer and Gavin Reid assemble contributors including teachers, psychologists and eminent researchers, offering guidance and insight into the range of challenges and possible solutions. In Chapter One, the editors highlight the needs of multilingual children, their parents and communities, stressing the importance of preserving different cultures whilst ensuring equality of educational opportunities. They examine the key factors influencing the education of multilingual learners with dyslexia and provide an overview of the rest of the book. Further chapters cover identification, assessment and teaching approaches, stressing the need to understand the language, culture and context of different countries and the differences between dyslexic monolingual and dyslexic multilingual students. Important links are made between assessment and teaching. Practical teaching approaches are detailed, including the value of ICT in classroom practice.

Chapters relating to policy and interventions take a more 'macro' overview, considering issues which need to be dealt with by managers and policy makers, particularly racism, in the light of the MacPherson report. Final sections address post-school aspects of multilingualism and also the considerable difficulties that additional language learning can present for children and adults with dyslexia. The style and quality of these international contributions vary. However, this is a book that a reader can 'dip into' as required. It will interest parents, teachers and policy makers, and provide a valuable source of reference to students. The editors suggest that the concept of inclusive education should encompass this group of learners, and this theme runs throughout the book. This book deserves a wide readership. It is hoped through this, the needs of multilingual young people with literacy difficulties will receive more focused attention and appropriate provision.

Judith Jones, Inspector-Adviser (Special Educational Needs), City of Salford.

Publications - Editor's choice

A number of publications have reached my attention this year, and these are just a few of the highlights.

Dyslexia and Information and Communications Technology - A Guide for Teachers and parents by Anita Keates, 2000, David Fulton Publishers

It is never easy to write a book in an areas that is changing so rapidly, but Anita Keates has drawn upon years of experience, much of it in the BDA Dyslexia Computer Committee, to provide teachers with an excellent resource designed to enable them to provide ICT support to dyslexics and maximise access to the National Curriculum.

Individual Education Plans - Dyslexia

by Janet Todd, 2000, David Fulton Publishers
Most teachers would agree that the good IEP holds the key to a successful intervention programme. This book provides details on how to create an ongoing teaching and learning programme, without being patronising or prescriptive. It offers background, ideas, and a way forward to build IEPs for you own specific needs, and ensure a whole school approach is implemented.

Understanding Developmental Dyspraxia - A textbook for students and professionals by Madeleine Portwood, 2000, David Fulton Publishers

When looking at the 'whole child' it is always important to understand that one area should not be investigated in isolation from others, particularly when they have overlapping diagnostic criteria. This book is an authoritative review of dyspraxia by one of the leading practitioners, and will no doubt appear on many recommended read lists very soon.

Dyslexia in Practice - A guide for teachers by Janet Townend and Martin Turner, 2000, Kluwer Academic/Plenum Publishers

This book provides an background for any teacher wishing to come to grips with the ideas behind implementation of a successful remediation programme. It helps the teacher to have a deeper understanding of the linguistic and cognitive difficulties of the child, from which they may build an informed intervention programme.

Dyslexics I Have Known: Reaching for the Stars by Bevé Hornsby, 2000,Whurr

So much of what is now available for dyslexics can be traced back to the work of Bevé Hornsby, her pioneering work at the Hornsby Centre and her books such as Alpha to Omega. This book is a mixture of insightful comment, personal record, and discussions of good practice, all of which are wonderful comments. For those who have been fortunate enough to cross her path, they will know what I mean when I say this book is "very Bevé!"

Teaching Children to Think by Robert Fisher, 1995, Stanley Thornes

Although this is not a new book, it was only recently that I had an opportunity to read it. I believe it is an excellent introduction to the rich area of teaching that is still relatively under explored, namely the development of children's ability to become independent thinkers. It covers creative thinking, critical thinking, problem solving, instrumental enrichment and philosophy in a brief but informative way. All of these are extremely useful areas to develop for the dyslexic individual.

Publications list

• All prices include handling and postage within UK.

• The year indicates the most recent edition.

1. GENERAL INFORMATION.

Dyslexia Contact.

Official Magazine of the British Dyslexia Association. Published three times a year. Available only to BDA members and subscribers. (See G06 mailing list.)

Dyslexia Friendly Schools Pack. BDA. (2000) £5.00

For school orders on headed notepaper, special rate £2 only to cover p&p.

Eight fact-sheets in a folder, Foreword by David Blunkett. Good practice in school policy, tips for classroom teachers, liaison with parents, signs of dyslexia, comments by dyslexics about their school experiences and sources of further information.

Dyslexia: Early Help, Better Future. Augur, J. BDA (1998) £2.50

Early recognition of dyslexia is vital if children are to be provided with the special help they need to cope with school. A guide to signs that can help to identify a dyslexic child before school age, and the practical steps that can be taken.

Music and Dyslexia. BDA Music & Dyslexia Committee. BDA (1996) £1.50

Musical difficulties associated with dyslexia and practical suggestions. Guidelines for the Examining of Dyslexic Candidates from the Associated Board of the Royal Schools of Music.

This Book Doesn't Make Sense. Augur, J. Whurr (1995) £13.50

By Jean Augur, former BDA Education Director, teacher and parent. The book summarises the author's home and classroom experiences and includes practical advice on how to help and encourage dyslexic people to develop their full potential.

2. PARENTS

The Role of the Educational Psychologist in Assessment and Diagnosis. BDA (1997) £2.50

An invaluable guide for the parent whose child may be dyslexic. Describes the key role of the Educational Psychologist in assessment and diagnosis, and the tests used. Helpful advice for the parent involved in the assessment process.

Survival Kit: Preventing Parental Burn-out. Peer. L. BDA (1997) £1.50

Practical advice on taking action and controlling the inevitable personal stress involved in bringing up dyslexic children.

A Young Person's Guide to Dyslexia. Peer. L. BDA (1997) £1.50

To be read to the young person by a teacher or a parent and used as a discussion document. An aid to the classroom teacher when explaining Dyslexia/Specific Learning Difficulties, it may help in making pupils aware of dyslexia and more understanding and supportive towards dyslexic classmates.

Seven Ways to Help Your Child with Reading. Geere, B. £4.50

Seven Ways to Help Your Child with Maths. Geere, B. £4.50

Two booklets produced for all that provide practical suggestions for stimulating interest in reading and maths through everyday examples, games and activities.

Take Time. Nash-Wortham, M. And Hunt, J. (1997) £10.95

One root cause of difficulties with reading, writing or spelling can be a lack of co-ordination, rhythm and timing. This book brings movement and speech together in a series of short, regular exercises that help develop a child's concentration, confidence and balance. For parents, teachers and therapists.

3. EDUCATION

Information on Dyslexia for Primary Schools. BDA (1995) £2.50

Concise outline of the nature of dyslexia and the obligations of schools towards children with special educational needs for teachers, governors and all school staff.

Dyslexia in Primary Schools: Assessment into Action. (2nd Edition) BDA (2000) £7.50

For primary teachers who want help with dyslexic children in mainstream schools. Dyslexia specialists offer practical advice from their experience. This revised edition has two new chapters relating to working with dyslexic learners in the Literacy and Numeracy Strategies.

Winning with Dyslexia. A Guide for Secondary Schools. (3rd Edition) Peer, L. BDA (2000) £7.50

Every dyslexic student has different difficulties and needs.

This practical guide to secondary school life addresses the full range of issues, from building literacy to study skills and the use of computers.

Multilingualism, Literacy and Dyslexia: A Challenge for the Educators. Peer, L. and Reid, G. David Fulton Publishers with BDA. (2000) £19.50

An invaluable reference on assessment and support for bilingual learners and those needing to acquire a modern foreign language. It is an essential text for staff development. Reference is made to innovative approaches in technology and other teaching programmes beneficial to multilingual learners and those learning additional languages.

Day to Day Dyslexia in the Classroom. Pollock, J. and Waller, E. Routledge (1997) £14.50

Invaluable advice, written in jargon-free language, on how teachers can recognise specific learning difficulties and give practical help to develop the language, literacy and numeracy skills of affected children in their classes.

English Grammar and Teaching Strategies. Lifeline to Literacy. Pollock, J. and Waller, E. David Fulton Publishers. (1999) £12.00

This book aims to demystify grammar and equip any teacher to teach it in the class-room. Each grammatical item is clearly defined. Varieties of usage are illustrated.

Teaching Today Pack: Dyslexia in the Primary School (Video & Booklet) BBC (1997) Available only from BBC Educational Publishing, PO Box 234, Wetherby, W Yorks, LS23 7EU. Price £29.99 + £2 p&p.

The video and detailed booklet, produced by the BBC for the BDA, will help the primary school teacher to identify, understand and give practical support to the child with specific learning difficulties. The video sets out practical methods for identifying and teaching the dyslexic child in the mainstream primary classroom, and the booklet documents the range of techniques and resources that can be used.

4. SPECIALIST INFORMATION

Dyslexia: A Guide for the Medical Profession. Carlisle, J. BDA (1996) £1.50

Basic information on the condition for general practitioners, health visitors and other medical professions. This will enable them to assist in the early recognition of dyslexia and to recommend appropriate support and assistance for affected children and their families.

5. COMPUTER PUBLICATIONS

C18 Communicating in writing. Stansfield, J. BDA (Oct 1998) £4.50.

This booklet explains software and hardware (including portables) for word-processing, spell-checking and keyboard skills. It is helpful for dyslexic users to understand the range of possibilities and to choose what is best for individual needs.

Voice Activated Software and Futuristic Technology: The Way Ahead. Collated by Cotgrove, A. and Draffan, E.A.B., BDA (2000) £7.00

Information for practitioners about using the latest technologies to support dyslexic learners.

"Catch 'em Young". Stansfield, J. REM & BDA (Jul 2000) £7.00.

A valuable asset to anyone involved in the support of very young children who may be dyslexic. It is full of ideas and suggestions for the use of technology to support these young learners.

Dyslexia and Information Communications Technology. A Guide for Teachers and Parents. Keates, A. David Fulton (Publishers) Ltd. (Jan. 2000) £14.50.

Practical and accessible advice for teachers keen to enhance their dyslexic pupils' access to the curriculum through the use of ICT. Achievable goals for ICT novices and for more advanced users. It will help parents to understand and support their child's specific learning difficulty.

5th BDA International Conference

DYSLEXIA:
At the dawn of the new century

University of York
18-21 April 2001

"It is with very great pleasure that we invite you to join us at the prestigious 5th International Conference organised by the British Dyslexia Association where there will be over 250 papers, posters and workshops. As ever it is a platform for debate and investigation into research, effective practice, new innovations and policy. It is the forum at which current and future needs of the widest order will be discussed by a broad range of international experts. A contribution to these debates by all attendees is both needed and highly valued.

"We look forward to seeing you in the beautiful and historic City of York in April 2001 and sharing the dynamics of a conference that will most definitely be looking into provision for the changing needs of dyslexic people at the Dawn of the New Century."

Lindsay Peer, Education Director, BDA
Professor Rod Nicolson, Conference Chair

Checkout the full programme at:
www.bdainternationalconference.org

Index of advertisers